CHAIR YOGA FOR SENIORS

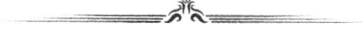

The Illustrated Guide to
Achieve Better Mobility,
Flexibility & Fitness with Easy
Stress-Free Exercises in Just
10 Minutes a Day

MOVEMENT FREEDOM PUBLICATIONS

CONTENTS

To my community at The Villages, Florida—thank you for welcoming me into your lives and allowing me the privilege of serving you.

To my beloved grandmother, whose strength, perseverance, and love for movement continue to inspire me. Your determination to stay active despite life's challenges was a powerful reminder that movement is life. This book is a tribute to you and the lessons you taught me.

To every senior seeking strength, balance, and vitality—this book is for you. Amidst a full work week, motherhood, marriage, and service, I poured my heart into this guide because I believe in your ability to heal, strengthen, and thrive. May it bring you movement, freedom, and joy.

Lastly, to my Creator—Thank You for placing this passion in my heart, walking with me through every step, and leading me to serve others through healing and movement.

"Refuse to lay down your spirit. Refuse to let your body fade. Movement is Life—Get Moving."

— DR YVETTE F.

INTRODUCTION

"The best time to plant a tree was 20 years ago. The second-best time is now."

— CHINESE PROVERB

"Don't grow old!" is a phrase I hear almost daily working with senior patients. If anyone has witnessed aging at its best —and at its worst—it's me. In my published guide, *Top Ten Benefits of Orthopedic Physical Therapy for Seniors,* I highlight the benefits of this specialized practice, as I use evidence-based strategies to address age-related changes like loss of balance, strength, flexibility, and stamina. Many readers have contacted me to share how transitioning to a home-based wellness program after completing their physical therapy program has been empowering and life-supporting. They continue to move confidently and return to active daily routines. I believe in the power of effective, age-appropriate, and well-designed exercise programs and am passionate about doing my part to produce and share them with those who can benefit the most.

I currently lead a skilled orthopedic physical therapy team in The Villages, Florida, and we live for the moments when our senior patients graduate from their therapy programs to a tailored wellness plan. Our clinic lights up as staff and patients cheer and announce, "We have a graduate in the house!" Our mission is to empower patients to continue making and managing progress independently.

This book aims to help you achieve the same sense of accomplishment and success through a safe, effective, science-backed daily home exercise routine.

How Is This Chair Yoga Book Different?

As a Doctor of Physical Therapy with over 23 years of experience working with seniors, I deeply understand the physical and mental challenges that come with aging. I've seen how a sedentary lifestyle accelerates decline while consistent movement slows it. I know the mental and emotional struggle many seniors face when their minds tell them they can still move like they did years ago, but their bodies refuse to cooperate.

I've seen seniors stop moving due to fear—whether it's fear of falling or fear of pain—only to find that these fears become self-fulfilling. The phrase 'Use it or lose it' rings true: avoiding movement increases your risk of both pain and injury. Avoiding movement leads to **muscle weakness, joint stiffness, and decreased circulation**, which in turn makes everyday activities feel even more difficult. Over time, this inactivity can cause a decline in balance and coordination, increasing the very risks—falls and pain—that many seniors were trying to avoid in the first place.

This book is not just another chair yoga guide. It's a thoughtfully crafted, evidence-based resource designed to help seniors move safely and effectively. Every pose portrayed in these 10-minute routines is intentionally selected with the senior age group in mind to yield the best physical results with the lowest risk of injury or discomfort. By following the 10-minute daily routines in this book, you can expect to see physical improvements within two to four weeks.

Initially, the poses may feel challenging or uncomfortable, but they will become more effortless and more fluid over time. The expectation is that the mobility, flexibility, and strength you will gain after habitually doing these routines will translate to greater ease with everyday activities such as standing, walking, bending, and even preventing falls. For seniors in the early stages of physical decline, these routines may help restore confidence and enjoyment in recreational activities. For those with multiple health issues, medical challenges, or significant loss of body strength, these routines are a good starting point to get back into movement and exercise, focusing on returning to daily independent activities. Regardless of your current level of fitness, the focus of these routines is to promote, elevate, and maintain your best physical quality of life.

Unlike many other chair yoga books, I've also included a bonus: a **Functional Movement Screen** that evaluates your strength, balance, and mobility. This tool helps determine your current physical level and injury risk, allowing you to tailor the program safely and effectively to your capabilities. Starting an exercise routine without this understanding can lead to injury, something I've seen too often in my work.

Aging Is Inevitable, but Decline Is Not

My grandma passed away at the age of 95. We were very close, and reflecting on her life still brings tears to my eyes. She remained physically independent until her mid-80s when arthritis began affecting her hip. Like many older adults, she instinctively started avoiding movements that caused pain, which only made her hip progressively stiffer.

The routine I designed for her emphasized gentle core activation, targeted stretches, and gradual strengthening exercises to promote flexibility and stability without exacerbating pain. By staying consistent with these targeted movements, she was able to reduce stiffness and regain more natural, pain-free movement. I also explained to my family that keeping her active was essential. However, they naturally wanted to prioritize her comfort, which often meant encouraging rest. While this instinct is understandable, it can lead to unintended consequences.

When we stop using specific muscles and joints, they weaken and stiffen. Compensatory movements—such as shifting weight differently—can cause imbalances that lead to further discomfort. The only way to prevent this is to practice these types of movements so they are not lost altogether.

Grandma made a proactive choice: She decided to keep moving. Through daily exercises and encouragement, she stayed engaged in activities she loved—gardening, cooking (she made the best fried chicken!), and even dancing with her grandchildren. Her determination was and is a powerful reminder that **movement is life**. Gentle, consistent movement can slow the aging process, preserving not only physical health but also joy and quality of life.

Many seniors face similar challenges, and their responses typically fall into one of three categories:

1. They **give in** to their physical limitations and stop doing the activities they love.
2. They **disregard** their limitations and push through, risking further injury.
3. They **thoughtfully address** their limitations, finding safe ways to stay active.

Aging is universal, but how we navigate it depends on our choices. By adopting mindful movement practices, we can build resilience and improve both mobility and strength. The human body can adapt and grow stronger at any age when given the right tools. With consistent effort, mindful, mechanically sound movement can slow decline and restore confidence in daily activities.

Who Is This Book For?

This guide is for you if:

- You've completed physical therapy and want to maintain your progress.
- You've had an orthopedic procedure and need a safe way to rebuild strength and mobility.
- You're experiencing physical challenges that make daily activities more difficult.
- You live alone and want to stay independent and confident.
- You're a caregiver or family member of a senior who needs better mobility and safety.

This book provides practical, evidence-based guidance on how to build strength, flexibility, and balance through chair yoga. Each chapter offers clear instructions, gentle encouragement, and simple, actionable steps to create a sustainable daily movement routine.

Why Chair Yoga?

Chair yoga is an ideal exercise choice for those who need a safe, adaptable alternative to traditional workouts. It focuses on gentle movements that minimize joint strain while improving strength, flexibility, and balance. It is especially beneficial for individuals with conditions such as osteoporosis, arthritis, general deconditioning, or those recovering from hip replacements, as it offers gentle movement without compromising safety.

The guidance throughout this book blends classic yoga poses and modified poses used in physical therapy settings into safe, accessible movements performed while seated in a stable chair. Exercising while sitting eliminates the fear of falling and reduces strain on sensitive joints, making it perfect for individuals with arthritis, mobility limitations, or balance concerns.

Chair yoga's greatest strength is its adaptability, allowing people with varying physical needs to engage safely and effectively. Whether managing chronic conditions, recovering from an injury, or simply seeking a gentle way to stay active, chair yoga meets you where you are. It can improve strength, posture, core stability, and balance—all from the comfort of a sturdy chair.

My Experience and Commitment

I've worked with countless seniors facing mobility challenges, chronic pain, and post-surgical recovery. I've seen how movement transforms lives physically, emotionally, and mentally. This book is born from that experience.

Common questions I hear are, "I've finished physical therapy —now what?", "I'm not ready for a gym, but I must keep moving. What could I do?" or "I've played pickleball for years. Why are my legs giving out on me? Why did I fall?". I am deeply passionate about offering reliable and practical solutions to bridge that gap.

Throughout my career, I've gained a deep understanding of the challenges seniors face—joint degeneration, muscle stiffness, balance loss, and the emotional toll of feeling physically limited. However, these challenges don't have to define your life. With the right approach, you can regain confidence, reduce pain, and embrace daily activities with energy and ease.

Words of Wisdom: You might feel, in your mind, that you can still move like you did 20 or 30 years ago, but your body may not cooperate. It's easy to flare up an arthritic joint or lose your balance. Walking the golf course, hitting a pickleball, or bending to release a bowling ball may now feel more brutal. The good news is that specific daily exercises can **slow physical aging**, keeping you active, confident, and safer from injury. Keep reading, and you will learn the best exercise routines to start making positive changes.

A Note on Safety

This book provides adaptable exercises, but you must consult your physician before starting any new fitness routine, especially if you have underlying health conditions. Listen to your body, take breaks as needed, and modify poses, breaths, and repetitions to suit your abilities.

Let's embark on this journey toward better health, greater independence, and renewed vitality together.

Welcome to your chair yoga journey!

1

UNDERSTANDING CHAIR YOGA AND ITS BENEFITS

"Take care of your body. It's the only place you have to live."

— JIM ROHN

Years ago, I had two clients, George and Jim, both dealing with lower back pain from arthritis. George loved golfing and gardening, while Jim led a more sedentary lifestyle. Despite their similar conditions, their recoveries were very different. George had been practicing chair yoga, which kept his body flexible and strong. He progressed steadily and regained confidence in his movements. Jim, however, struggled due to stiffness and deconditioning, making his recovery much slower.

This experience reveals a valuable lesson: regular, gentle movement like chair yoga can significantly improve recovery and help seniors stay resilient and active.

WHAT IS CHAIR YOGA? A GENTLE INTRODUCTION

Chair yoga adapts traditional yoga poses for practice while seated or using a chair for support. By removing the challenge of balancing while standing, chair yoga allows you to safely focus on movement and alignment. For those with back issues or joint discomfort, chair yoga provides an accessible way to gain the benefits of exercise without the fear of aggravating pre-existing conditions.

Yoga originated in ancient India as a spiritual and physical discipline. Over the centuries, it has evolved to meet the needs of diverse populations. Chair yoga emerged as an innovative adaptation, making yoga accessible to people with mobility challenges, chronic conditions, or injury recovery. Today, it is embraced in senior centers, rehabilitation facilities, and homes worldwide.

But chair yoga is more than just physical exercise. It offers a holistic approach to well-being, addressing the mind, body, and spirit. Physically, it strengthens muscles, improves flexibility, and supports balance. Mentally, it reduces stress, sharpens focus, and enhances mood. Emotionally, it fosters connection and reduces feelings of isolation, especially in group settings.

Chair yoga is truly for everyone—seniors managing arthritis, individuals recovering from injuries, or anyone seeking a gentle yet effective exercise routine. Its adaptability ensures that no matter your starting point, there's a place for you in chair yoga.

THE SCIENCE BEHIND CHAIR YOGA: HEALTH BENEFITS FOR SENIORS

Chair yoga's physical benefits are profound. It gently counteracts joint stiffness and loss of flexibility through low-impact movements. Each pose stretches and strengthens muscles, enhancing overall mobility while supporting safe movement.

Studies have shown that chair yoga can significantly improve functional fitness and reduce pain levels among seniors. These benefits translate into easier daily activities, such as bending down to tie shoes or reaching for items on a high shelf.

Regular chair yoga practice also improves balance and coordination. Simple, repetitive movements train the body to respond to shifts in weight and position, reducing the risk of falls. Improved balance fosters confidence in daily movements, creating a sense of security and ease.

Mentally, chair yoga serves as a powerful stress-reduction tool. Mindful breathing and focused movements calm the nervous system, reducing anxiety and enhancing mental clarity. This mind-body connection fosters emotional resilience, equipping you to handle daily challenges with a sense of calm.

Preventative health benefits are another cornerstone of chair yoga. Gentle stretching and strengthening exercises alleviate chronic pain, improve circulation, and reduce inflammation. Regular practice can also lessen dependency on pain medications.

Scientific studies have validated these benefits. Research on older adults with knee osteoarthritis found significant improvements in physical function and pain levels after 12 weeks of chair yoga. These findings highlight chair yoga's role as a safe, effective, and medication-free intervention for managing chronic conditions.

CHAIR YOGA VS. TRADITIONAL YOGA: KEY DIFFERENCES AND ADVANTAGES

Traditional yoga often includes standing and floor-based poses, which can be difficult for individuals with mobility limitations. Chair yoga adapts these movements in a seated position, reducing the risk of falls and joint strain. Reduced risk of injury makes chair yoga especially suitable for seniors, as it prioritizes safety and accommodates joint sensitivities.

One of chair yoga's greatest strengths is its versatility. It can be practiced almost anywhere—at home, in community centers, or even outdoors—making it easy to incorporate short, regular routines into daily life. This flexibility supports long-term health and vitality.

UNDERSTANDING SAFETY: HOW CHAIR YOGA PREVENTS INJURIES

Chair yoga is a gentle, low-impact form of exercise that helps prevent injuries in several ways:

1. Provides Stability and Support

- Using a **sturdy chair** reduces the risk of falls compared to standing yoga.
- **Controlled and grounded** movements make them safer for seniors with balance concerns.

2. Improves Strength and Flexibility

- **Gradual strengthening** of muscles, particularly in the **core, legs, and back**, helps improve stability and posture.
- **Gentle stretching** enhances flexibility, reducing muscle stiffness and preventing strains.

3. Enhances Body Awareness and Coordination

- Slow, mindful movements help seniors become

more aware of their body's position, reducing sudden, jerky movements that could cause injury.

- Repetitive movements **train coordination**, helping the body react better to balance challenges in daily life.

4. Reduces Joint Stress and Overuse Injuries

- Unlike high-impact exercises, chair yoga places **minimal strain on joints,** making it ideal for individuals with arthritis or joint pain.
- You can **modify movements** to avoid aggravating existing conditions.

5. Encourages Proper Posture and Alignment

- Strengthening **postural muscles** helps prevent injuries related to poor posture, such as back pain or shoulder strain.
- Sitting in a **properly aligned position** supports the spine and reduces pressure on joints.

6. Prevents Falls and Improves Balance

- Seated balance exercises **train core stability,** which is crucial for preventing falls.
- Some movements **strengthen leg muscles,** improving the ability to stand and walk safely.

- Some movements strengthen arm muscles, improving the ability to **reach overhead** while remaining steady and sturdy through the trunk.

7. Promotes Gentle, Pain-Free Movements

- Chair yoga encourages **moving within a comfortable range of motion**, preventing overstretching or muscle strain.
- **Listen to your body** and avoid pushing into pain.

OVERCOMING FEAR: BUILDING CONFIDENCE TO START

Starting a new practice can feel intimidating, especially if you're concerned about injury or pain. I often ask my clients: *If you don't try, how will you know how it can help you? And if you don't act now, when and how will you improve your physical health?*

Your journey to make positive change starts now. Have confidence knowing that chair yoga is designed with safety in mind. The chair provides stability, and the gentle, controlled movements allow you to gradually build strength, flexibility, and confidence in your body.

The key is to start—but start small. Begin with short, manageable sessions, such as a 5-minute routine instead of 10 minutes. If needed, do fewer breaths and poses to ease into the practice. Focus on mastering one beginner-level routine at a time before progressing to intermediate ones. Celebrate small achievements—they are the building blocks of a strong foundation. With this solid base, you can safely advance toward becoming the best physical version of yourself.

Let your family and friends know you have committed to this journey. Lean on them for encouragement and allow them to celebrate your successes.

Final Thoughts

Chair yoga is one of the safest and most effective ways to add movement to your daily routine. It's designed to be **gentle, adaptable, and accessible**, making it an excellent choice for improving strength, flexibility, and confidence— no matter your starting point.

But chair yoga offers more than just physical benefits. It helps you develop **better balance, body awareness, and mindfulness**, all of which contribute to long-term mobility and independence. With each breath and movement, you're not just exercising—you're investing in your health, building resilience, and regaining control over how you move and feel.

Progress happens one step at a time. Start where you are, move at your own pace, and celebrate every small improvement. Over time, these simple movements will lead to greater strength, better posture, and improved overall well-being.

2

PREPARING FOR YOUR CHAIR YOGA JOURNEY

"You are never too old to set another goal or to dream a new dream."

— C.S. LEWIS

When you were a child, do you remember having a favorite spot to sit at home? Maybe it was a cozy chair where you'd relax and recharge. You likely had another chair for staying focused and productive, especially when tackling homework or projects. Each chair served a different purpose, shaping your mindset the moment you sat in it.

In the same way, the chair you choose for your yoga practice plays an important role. It should provide stability, comfort, and support while promoting the right mental state—calm, focused, and ready for movement. Selecting the right chair can help set the tone for a safe and rewarding session.

CHOOSING THE RIGHT CHAIR: SAFETY AND SUPPORT FIRST

Selecting the right chair is not just about comfort—it's about creating a foundation for safe and effective practice. Stability and sturdiness are essential. A wobbly or unstable chair can reduce focus and confidence and increase the risk of injury. Look for a chair with a solid frame, firm support, and a non-slip base to ensure safety during movement.

The height of your chair also plays a significant role in maintaining proper alignment. Your feet should rest flat on the ground, and your knees should form a 90-degree angle. This positioning supports good posture, prevents strain on your lower back, and allows you to engage your core effectively. If your chair is too high or too low, it can throw off your alignment and make poses uncomfortable or ineffective.

FEATURES TO LOOK FOR IN A YOGA CHAIR

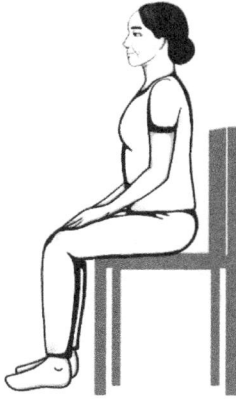

- **Stability:** Ensure the chair is sturdy and does not wobble.
- **Height:** Your feet should rest flat on the floor with knees at a 90-degree angle.
- **Non-Slip Feet:** Look for non-slip pads to prevent sliding.
- **No Wheels or Armrests:** Avoid chairs with wheels or bulky armrests that can obstruct movement.
- **Padding:** A cushioned seat can enhance comfort during longer sessions.

Standard dining room chairs often meet these criteria. Alternatively, yoga-specific chairs are designed for stability and can be an excellent investment for regular practice.

Tip: If you rely on armrests for support when sitting or standing, you can start with a chair with armrests and transition to an armless chair as your strength improves. Alternatively, position your chair near a sturdy table or countertop for extra support.

ESSENTIAL PROPS: TOOLS FOR ACCESSIBILITY AND COMFORT

Props in chair yoga are great assistive tools, especially for beginners. They support, stabilize, and enhance the practice and are especially beneficial for those with mobility concerns.

- **Yoga Blocks:** Use blocks to bring the ground closer during stretches or provide support under your feet.
- **Yoga Straps:** Straps help extend your reach and allow for deeper stretches without strain.
- **Cushions:** Add comfort to your seat or use them for lower back support.

Budget-Friendly Alternatives: Household items can serve as substitutes for traditional props:

- Use a rolled-up towel as a strap.
- Replace yoga blocks with sturdy books.
- Use a small pillow or cushion for added comfort.

ORGANIZING YOUR PROPS

Store your props in a basket or designated area near your practice space. Keeping them accessible prevents disruptions during your session and creates an inviting environment.

Creating a Safe Practice Space

Your chair yoga space should feel like a personal sanctuary—safe, uncluttered, and inviting. Consistency is key; practicing in the same space helps you establish a routine and make yoga an anticipated part of your day.

- **Clear the Area:** Remove loose rugs, cords, or other potential tripping hazards.
- **Adequate Lighting:** Natural light is ideal, but if that's not possible, ensure you have good artificial lighting.
- **Soothing Atmosphere:** Add plants, calming scents (e.g., lavender essential oil), or gentle background music.
- **Accessibility:** Ensure props and water are within easy reach.

These thoughtful touches transform your space into a peaceful retreat where you can focus on movement, breath, and mindfulness.

WHAT TO WEAR

Good chair yoga attire should prioritize **comfort, flexibility, and safety**, especially for seniors. Here are key recommendations:

1. Comfortable, Non-Restrictive Clothing

- **Loose-fitting or stretchable fabrics** (like cotton, bamboo, or moisture-wicking blends) allow for ease of movement.
- **Avoid tight or stiff clothing** that may restrict flexibility.
- **Layering is ideal** in case you get warm or cool during the session.

2. Supportive Footwear or Barefoot

- **Barefoot or non-slip socks** can provide better grip and connection with the floor.
- If shoes are preferred, **lightweight, flexible sneakers** with a non-slip sole can offer extra support.
- Avoid **heavy or rigid shoes** that could limit foot mobility.

3. Flexible Bottoms

4. Light layers like a zip-up jacket or shawl for warmth:

5. Optional Supportive Accessories

UNDERSTANDING YOUR BODY: LISTENING TO PAIN AND DISCOMFORT

Chair yoga is about honoring your body and its unique needs. Learning to differentiate between discomfort and pain is essential:

- **Discomfort:** Feelings of uneasiness when holding poses using weak muscles or stretching very tight muscles are normal and will reduce with gradual practice.
- **Pain:** Sharp or persistent pain is a signal to stop, reassess, and modify if possible.

Using a Pain Scale: On a scale of 0 to 10 (0 being no pain and 10 being severe pain), aim to stay below 5. If a pose causes discomfort beyond this level, adjust or choose a gentler variation.

Reflective Practice: After each session, note how your body feels. Write down any sensations, areas of tension, or improvements in flexibility.

COLLABORATING WITH HEALTHCARE PROVIDERS

If you have pre-existing medical conditions or physical limitations, consult your healthcare provider before beginning your chair yoga journey. A physical therapist or physician can offer personalized advice and ensure your practice supports your health needs.

If you have physical restrictions involving your arms or legs, focus on all other aspects of each routine that you can participate in. If you have physical restrictions involving your neck or your back, ensure you are seated with appropriate back support using a cushion. Engage in aspects of each routine that does not bring you discomfort or pain.

STARTING SLOW: BUILDING A SUSTAINABLE PRACTICE

Chair yoga is about creating a practice you can sustain over time, so start small and build as able:

- Build yourself up from 5-minute sessions to 10-minute sessions.
- Gradually increase the duration and complexity of your poses.
- Take breaks, listen to your body, and adjust for comfort.

Set Realistic Goals: Aim to practice consistently, whether it's three times a week or every day. Celebrate small milestones, such as ease with bending or reaching or the ability to sit up taller for longer periods. Keep a journal to track your progress and reflect on your journey.

Final Thoughts

Your chair yoga journey begins with thoughtful preparation —choosing the right chair, gathering simple props, creating a safe space, and tuning into your body. These foundational steps set the stage for a rewarding practice that nurtures your physical and mental well-being.

Take a deep breath, settle into your chair, and know that you're exactly where you need to be. The moment is here: This is your space, your time, and your opportunity to embrace movement, mindfulness, and self-care.

3

GETTING STARTED WITH CHAIR YOGA – FINDING YOUR STARTING POINT

"Believe you can, and you're halfway there."

— THEODORE ROOSEVELT

I n my physical therapy practice, every new patient begins with a **comprehensive evaluation** to determine their starting point. This includes assessing **strength, range of motion, flexibility, core stability, balance, and overall function**. Because no two individuals are the same, I develop a **personalized treatment plan** to help each patient progress toward their specific goals.

This book follows a similar approach. Before diving into the routines, it's important to **identify your starting level** so you can build a strong foundation and progress safely. Knowing where to begin will set you up for success and help you get the most out of your practice.

Now, let's get ready to **embark on this chair yoga journey!** Research shows that regular, gentle movement can significantly enhance both **physical and mental well-being**, making chair yoga an accessible and effective option for all. Whether you're a **complete beginner**, looking for guidance to **build on your progress**, or ready to **take on new challenges**, chair yoga meets you where you are.

This chapter will help you **determine your starting point** and explore three practice levels—**beginner, intermediate, and advanced**—so you can safely and confidently make chair yoga a part of your daily routine.

WHERE TO START: THREE STARTING POINTS

Beginner Level

This level is perfect for those who:

- Have never done chair yoga or traditional yoga.
- Have been recommended to start exercising but are not yet strong, safe, or confident enough to exercise while standing.
- Are dealing with conditions such as back or joint pain, arthritis, scoliosis, post-surgical limitations, a history of falling, weakness, incontinence, breathing

issues, stiffness, loss of mobility or flexibility, vertigo, or neuropathy.

- Have been sedentary and now find moving difficult.
- Recently graduated from an orthopedic physical therapy program, and want to implement chair yoga as a home exercise routine to maintain and build on their progress.

For beginners, chair yoga is an ideal choice to reintroduce exercise into your life. I have worked with many patients dealing with back pain and stiffness after years of sitting at a desk or playing sports, as well as many seniors recovering from knee, hip, or back surgery who are unsure how to stay active. I have seen how chair yoga can provide a gentle, adaptable way to build strength and regain control over posture and movements. As you establish your practice, you will:

- Feel stronger and more confident.
- Move with greater ease and flexibility.
- Breathe better and feel more energized.
- Begin to feel healthier as your efforts bring real, positive changes.

Intermediate Level

This level is designed for individuals who:

- May have some ailments or physical limitations but are generally independent and able to participate in daily routines without significant risk of injury.
- Need to take frequent breaks throughout the day and may only have the energy to exercise in short sessions.
- Experience some pain issues, but the pain is manageable and doesn't linger.
- Have some strength and endurance but are looking to build more.
- Want to try to return to physical or recreational activities.
- Are motivated to prevent a decline in their health and recognize that a sedentary lifestyle could lead to future problems.
- May live alone and are not confident about joining a gym or group class.

For intermediates, chair yoga can help you maintain independence and improve your physical abilities. With a daily routine, you can:

- Build on your existing strength and endurance.
- Improve your posture and balance.
- Boost your confidence and reduce the risk of injury.

- Prevent the health decline that often accompanies inactivity.

Advanced Level

This level is ideal for those who:

- Want to elevate their core strength, postural strength, stamina, and balance.
- Are independent in their daily activities and not significantly limited by pain.
- Are aware of their strengths and weaknesses and ready to push themselves further.
- Want to maintain or even improve their current level of function.
- May have emerging health concerns but are determined to stay physically strong and active.
- Have progressed from the beginner or intermediate levels and are now ready for more advanced challenges.

Advanced practitioners can use chair yoga to fine-tune their abilities and maintain their quality of life. By focusing on improving core strength, stamina, and balance, they can achieve greater physical resilience and begin or continue participating in activities they enjoy, such as softball, bowling, or pickleball. Chair yoga offers an opportunity to build on existing strengths while preventing future health challenges, ensuring a vibrant and active lifestyle. You can:

- Continue improving your strength, balance, and coordination.
- Prevent the impact of emerging health issues on your physical health.
- Celebrate your progress as you move beyond foundational exercises.

TRANSITIONING BETWEEN LEVELS

I recommend that everyone progress through this book's routines by moving from beginner to intermediate to advanced. You may find that at each level, some exercises may feel easy while others remain more challenging. That's perfectly normal. The key is to:

- Listen to your body and adapt your practice as needed.
- Mix and match exercises from different levels to create a routine that feels right for you.
- Be patient. Progress takes time and consistency, but each small step brings you closer to your goals.

Stay committed, and trust that your practice will continue to build strength, flexibility, and confidence.

Final Thoughts

Chair yoga is a journey; your starting point does not limit where you can go. With patience and dedication, you'll build strength, confidence, and a stronger connection to your body. No matter your experience level, I recommend beginning with the foundational routines to develop proper form and body awareness. From there, you can gradually progress to more advanced practices at your own pace, allowing your body to adapt and grow safely. Remember, each step forward is progress on the path to greater well-being.

4

FUNCTIONAL MOVEMENT SCREEN (BONUS 1)

"The secret of getting ahead is getting started."

— MARK TWAIN

I designed this Functional Movement Screen to give you a reliable idea of your current mobility, flexibility, strength, and balance. Determining this information before beginning your chair yoga practice is super helpful. By determining whether you fall into the Beginner, Intermediate, or Advanced level, you'll be better equipped to approach your practice safely, minimize the risk of injury, and build confidence in your abilities.

Instructions

- Perform each test slowly and with intention.
- Use a sturdy chair without wheels for stability.
- Have someone nearby for assistance or support if needed.
- Track your performance and compare your results with the scoring guidelines to identify your starting level.

MOVEMENT SCREEN TESTS

1. Seated Marching Test

Purpose: Assess hip flexibility, core stability, postural stability, and balance.

Instructions: Sit tall in your chair. Lift one knee up toward the ceiling, hold it for five seconds, and slowly lower it back down. Repeat with the opposite leg. Perform five repetitions per leg.

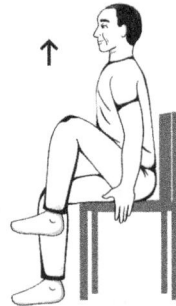

Scoring:

- **Beginner:** Difficulty lifting the knee above hip level or maintaining balance.

- **Intermediate:** Able to lift the knee comfortably and hold for five seconds with slight wobbling.
- **Advanced:** Easily lifts the knee and holds the position steadily for five seconds.

2. Seated Forward Bend

Purpose: Assess spine flexibility and hamstring mobility.

Instructions: Sit tall in your chair. Keep feet flat on the floor facing forward. Bend forward and reach down with both hands toward your toes.

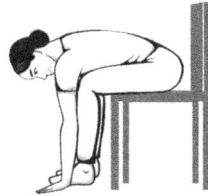

Scoring:

- **Beginner:** Able to reach only to the knees or shins.
- **Intermediate:** Able to reach the ankles with mild discomfort.
- **Advanced:** Comfortably able to touch toes or beyond.

3. Overhead Arm Reach

Purpose: Assess shoulder mobility and upper body flexibility and strength.

Instructions: Sit tall. Raise both arms overhead, keeping your elbows straight.

Scoring:

- **Beginner:** Unable to lift arms above ear level.
- **Intermediate:** Arms reach ear level but with noticeable stiffness, discomfort, or difficulty.
- **Advanced:** Arms fully extend overhead without discomfort.

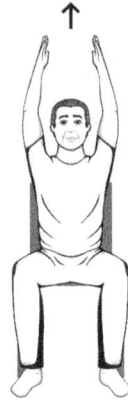

4. Seated Twist Test

Purpose: Assess spinal rotation mobility as well as neck and trunk flexibility.

Instructions: Sit tall. Place your right hand on the back of the chair and gently twist your torso to the left, looking over your shoulder. Hold the twist for five seconds. Repeat on the opposite side.

Scoring:

- **Beginner:** Minimal twist, difficulty holding position.
- **Intermediate:** Moderate twist, able to hold with slight discomfort.
- **Advanced:** Full twist, able to hold comfortably for five seconds both ways.

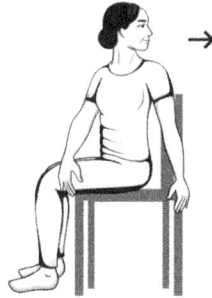

5. Seated Sit-to-Stand Test

Purpose: Assess leg strength, balance, and functional mobility.

Instructions: Sit at the edge of your chair with your feet flat on the ground. Raise your arms forward, then rise. Stand up fully if you can. Sit back down slowly. Perform five repetitions.

Scoring:

- **Beginner:** Unable to rise without using hands.
- **Intermediate:** Completes five reps with moderate effort. Occasionally uses hands for balance. Standing tall in between repetitions may feel challenging.

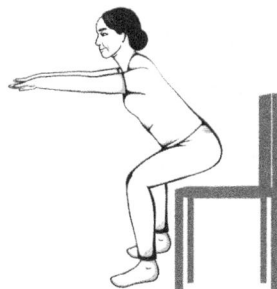

- **Advanced:** Completes five reps through full motion, hands-free, smoothly, and effortlessly.

SCORING YOUR MOVEMENT SCREEN

- **Beginner:** Scored "Beginner" on three or more tests.
- **Intermediate:** Scored "Intermediate" on three or more tests.
- **Advanced:** Scored "Advanced" on three or more tests.

Your results provide valuable insights into your current fitness level, guiding you to start at the most appropriate point in your chair yoga journey. Remember, progress is personal, and consistency will lead to improvement over time.

By identifying your functional movement level, you set yourself up for a safe, tailored, and effective chair yoga experience. Use this assessment as a foundation for growth and enjoy every step of your journey toward improved mobility, strength, and confidence!

5

UNDERSTANDING YOUR FUNCTIONAL MOVEMENT RESULTS

"The journey of a thousand miles begins with a single step."

— LAO TZU

Now that you've completed the Functional Movement Screen, it's time to interpret your results. This chapter will help you understand your starting level (Beginner, Intermediate, or Advanced) and provide tailored recommendations for beginning your chair yoga journey safely and effectively. Remember, these results are not meant to limit you but to empower you by confidently identifying where you can improve your strength, balance, and flexibility.

WHAT YOUR RESULTS MEAN

The Functional Movement Screen will help you determine which chair yoga starting level best suits your current abilities. Beginning at the appropriate level will reduce the risk of injury, build confidence, and allow you to experience steady progress.

Beginner Level

If you scored "Beginner" on three or more tests:

- You may have physical limitations such as joint pain, stiffness, or limited mobility.
- Daily activities may feel challenging or require additional support.
- You may feel hesitant about movement due to fear of pain or falling.

Recommendation: Start with the Beginner Chair Yoga routines. Focus on building foundational strength, core stability, and flexibility. Gradually increase your endurance as you gain confidence. The key is to take it slow and celebrate small victories along the way.

Intermediate Level

If you scored "Intermediate" on three or more tests:

- You have some mobility and strength but may experience occasional discomfort or fatigue.
- You can perform daily activities with moderate effort but may require breaks.
- You may have mild stiffness or balance issues but can move independently.

Recommendation: Begin with Intermediate Chair Yoga routines. These routines will help you maintain independence, improve balance, and enhance core strength. Pay attention to any areas of discomfort and adjust poses as needed to prevent overexertion.

Advanced Level

If you scored "Advanced" on three or more tests:

- You have adequate core stability, mobility, and balance.
- You can perform most daily activities without significant difficulty.
- You are motivated to push your limits and improve your physical performance.

Recommendation: Start with Advanced Chair Yoga routines to challenge your core, balance, and stamina. Focus on refining your movements, enhancing posture, and maintaining your current fitness level. Advanced routines will keep your body resilient and prepared for a wide range of activities.

TAILORING YOUR PRACTICE

Regardless of your starting level, chair yoga will grow with you. Progression isn't always linear, and you will find that certain poses feel easier while others present a challenge. Here are some strategies to personalize your practice:

- **Adjust Intensity:** Modify the depth of stretches or duration of poses to match your comfort level.
- **Incorporate Props:** Use blocks, straps, or cushions to support your body and enhance your alignment.
- **Track Your Progress:** Keep a journal to record improvements, areas of difficulty, and milestones achieved.

REASSESSING OVER TIME

As you continue your chair yoga journey, it's essential to periodically reassess your abilities. Repeating the Functional Movement Screen every few months can help you track your progress and adjust your practice accordingly.

Signs that it's time to reassess:

- You find beginner or intermediate routines too easy and are ready for a greater challenge.
- Your flexibility, balance, or strength has noticeably improved.
- You feel more confident and capable during daily activities that used to be difficult.

OVERCOMING COMMON CHALLENGES

Don't be discouraged if your results are lower than you expected. It doesn't take much for muscles to lose strength or size. Research indicates that muscle atrophy can commence rapidly during periods of immobility, with measurable losses occurring within just a few days. A period of immobility could be an overnight stay at the hospital or a few days of not doing much due to having a cold or the flu. In any case, it is better to start any new exercise program cautiously and progress to higher levels gradually for optimal safety and success.

Strategies for Overcoming Obstacles:

- **Start Small:** Focus on one pose at a time. Gradual improvement leads to long-term success.
- **Seek Support:** Engage with a yoga instructor, physical therapist, or online community for advice and encouragement.

- **Be Patient:** Progress may be slow, but consistency is key. Trust the process and celebrate every improvement.

SAFETY AND SELF-CARE

Your safety is the top priority. Chair yoga is designed to be gentle and supportive, but if you are experiencing any difficulty, it is important to listen to your body and take breaks when needed.

Tips for Safe Practice:

- Warm up with gentle movements before starting your routine.
- Maintain good posture to protect your back and joints.
- Stay hydrated and rest if you feel fatigued or lightheaded.
- Avoid pushing through pain. Modify or skip poses that cause discomfort.
- Complete the cool-downs at the end of the routines.

Final Thoughts

Your Functional Movement Screen results are a starting point on your path to improved mobility, strength, and balance. Beginning your chair yoga journey at the suggested level will better equip you to succeed. Remember that progress is unique to each individual—honor your body, trust your journey, and celebrate every step forward.

Let's continue this journey toward greater well-being in the next chapter. In it, you'll learn my 'center-out' approach to building strength and stability from the center of the body, branching out to the limbs.

6

FULL BODY STRENGTH STARTS WITH CENTERED STABILITY

"Energy flows where intention goes."

— JAMES REDFIELD

Now that you've identified your starting level, it's time to set yourself up for success! In my physical therapy practice, I prioritize strengthening and stabilizing the center of the body before strengthening the arms and legs. The center of the body involves muscles that stabilize and support the pelvic floor organs and the spine. Lack of adequate muscle strength in these areas can result in musculoskeletal issues, including incontinence, poor posturing, and loss of balance control. When movement becomes unstable, injury risk rises.

I am happy to share that this center-focused approach has also been a cornerstone of traditional yoga. In this chapter, we'll learn the yoga ways and draw a parallel with my way. For the best safety and comfort, I recommend engaging and maintaining activation of these muscle groups before holding yoga poses and during any movement transitions.

STRENGTHENING FROM THE CENTER OUT: THE ROLE OF BANDHAS

In yoga, Bandhas refer to internal muscular engagements that promote physical stability and control. Bandhas involve three key areas of engagement:

- **Pelvic Floor Engagement (Mula Bandha)**
- **Core Muscle Engagement (Uddiyana Bandha)**
- **Postural Alignment (Jalandhara Bandha)**

These engagements help to:

- Strengthen essential stabilizing muscles.
- Support proper posture.
- Enhance balance and mobility.
- Reduce the risk of falls and injuries.

The sections below explain each area in practical terms, emphasizing how they support stability, balance, and functional movement.

PRACTICAL APPLICATIONS OF BANDHAS IN CHAIR YOGA

1. Pelvic Floor Engagement (Mula Bandha)

Location: Pelvic floor muscles at the base of the spine.

How to Engage: Gently contract the pelvic floor muscles, similar to stopping the flow of urine (commonly known as a Kegel). You should feel a tightening and lifting sensation at the base of the pelvis. Maintain this contraction while breathing naturally.

Benefits:

- Strengthens the pelvic floor, helping to prevent issues such as urinary incontinence and pelvic organ prolapse.
- Works with core and postural muscles to create a stable center.

Application in Chair Yoga: Engage the pelvic floor during all assertive poses to enhance pelvic and spinal stability.

2. Core Muscle Engagement (Uddiyana Bandha)

Location: Lower abdominal region, specifically the transverse abdominis (deepest abdominal muscle).

How to Engage: Exhale fully, then gently draw your abdomen inward and slightly upward, moving your navel toward your spine. Maintain this engagement while breathing naturally.

Benefits:

- Stabilizes the spine and reduces back strain.
- Acts as an internal back brace. When engaged, it tightens around the lower trunk, protecting the spine and improving posture.

Application in Chair Yoga: Engage the core *and* pelvic floor muscles simultaneously during assertive poses to support spinal alignment and stability.

3. Upper Body Postural Alignment – Chin Tucks (Jalandhara Bandha)

Location: Neck and throat area.

How to Engage: Gently tuck the chin toward the chest by moving the base of the head backward while lifting the sternum, keeping the shoulders relaxed.

Benefits:

- Corrects forward head posture.
- Supports upper spinal and shoulder stability.
- Supports overhead reaching and upright balance.

Application in Chair Yoga: Perform chin tucks during poses involving neck or arm movements to maintain proper alignment.

4. Mid-trunk Postural Alignment – Back Squeezes (Scapular Retractions)

Location: Upper-mid back area.

How to Engage: Sit tall and pull your shoulder blades inward and downward as if pinching them together while lifting the sternum. Avoid lifting or hiking your shoulders.

Benefits:

- Improves spinal posture and shoulder alignment.
- Enhances neck and arm movement.
- Opens the lungs, supporting full breaths.

Application in Chair Yoga: Perform scapular retractions alongside chin tucks during poses that involve raising or reaching with the arms.

INTEGRATING THESE PRINCIPLES: BUILDING
STABILITY IN SEATED MOUNTAIN POSE

Follow these steps to improve the engagement of your pelvic floor, core, and postural muscles effectively in the Seated Mountain Pose:

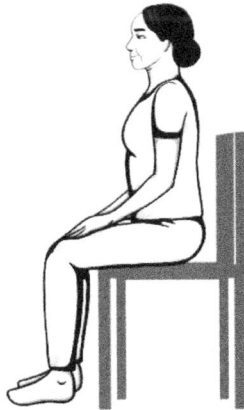

1. **Sit Tall:** Sit in a sturdy chair with your feet flat on the floor. Place your hands on your thighs and lengthen your spine. Contract the lower muscles first, then move upward.
2. **Pelvic Floor Engagement:** Contract the pelvic floor muscles as if stopping the flow of urine. Hold for 2-3 breaths, then release.
3. **Core Engagement:** Draw your abdomen inward and slightly upward, moving your navel toward your spine. Maintain this engagement for 2-3 breaths.

4. **Scapular Retractions:** Pull your shoulder blades inward. Keep your upper shoulders relaxed, and avoid hiking them. Hold each pinch for 2-3 breaths.

5. **Chin Tucks:** Gently tuck your chin while lifting your sternum, ensuring proper head and neck alignment. Hold for 2-3 breaths, then release.

6. **Combine All Engagements:** Engage all four muscle groups simultaneously for 2-3 breaths, focusing on posture and steady breathing.

If these principles are new to you, I recommend you practice the above sequence regularly, repeating each muscular engagement individually and simultaneously three times daily to build a strong foundation of stability. The control you develop will enhance your chair yoga routines and be instrumental in reducing spinal, pelvic, and balance issues.

WHY THESE PRINCIPLES MATTER FOR SENIORS

- **Pelvic Floor and Core Stability:** Most of our senior clients show loss of muscle control and strength in these areas, contributing to commonly diagnosed back pain, fall risk, and urinary incontinence.
- **Postural Control:** Many older clients with neck, shoulder, and balance issues have difficulty demonstrating good upper body and head posturing due to weakness, stiffness, and pain.

- **Prevention of Age-Related Conditions:** Consistent engagement of these postural, core, and pelvic floor muscle groups reduces the risk of the above conditions and allows for comfortable participation with progressed chair yoga.
- **Mind-Body Connection:** Integrating these engagements with mindful breathing fosters mental clarity, emotional balance, and physical well-being.

Final Thoughts

By focusing on these foundational principles, you can transform your chair yoga practice into a powerful tool for improving stability, mobility, and overall wellness. Consistent practice will make these muscular engagements second nature, empowering you to move with confidence and ease.

7

CHAIR YOGA POSE LIBRARY

"With each movement, we uncover strength we didn't know we had."

— ANONYMOUS

Chair yoga is a versatile and accessible way to enhance strength, flexibility, and balance at any age. This chapter provides a detailed guide to the carefully selected poses used throughout this book, categorized by skill level: all levels, intermediate, and advanced. Each selected pose serves a function- to improve commonly seen age-related physical decline. I use these poses and programs with my senior clients and have had a high success rate in helping them return to higher levels of function and movement freedom. Use this library to familiarize yourself with the poses and build confidence before progressing to the routines.

SECTION 1: SEATED POSES FOR ALL LEVELS

These foundational poses are safe, effective, and suitable for beginners. If you have not developed your pelvic floor, core, and postural stability, I recommend you start here. These poses focus on alignment, gentle movement, controlled engagement, and relaxation to build confidence and body awareness. The goal is to hold each pose for 2 to 3 breaths. It is okay to start with holding a pose for 1-breath and gradually build to longer holds when able.

1. Mountain Pose

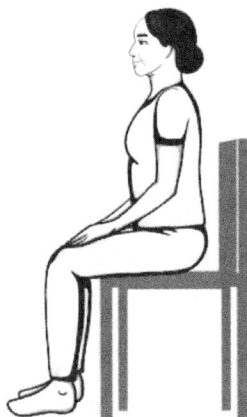

Purpose: Improves posture, engages core and pelvic muscles, and allows focused breathwork.

Instructions: Sit tall with your feet flat on the floor and your knees aligned over your ankles. Lengthen your spine and rest your hands on your thighs.

At rest: You are facing forward, arms and legs relaxed, focusing on breathing in through your nose fully then out through your nose or pursed lips fully. Each full breath amounts to about five seconds. Practice progressing from 1-breath holds to up to 3-breath holds.

Engagements: In the same position, you are engaging your pelvic floor muscles and core, lifting your chest, squeezing your shoulder blades together, and finishing with a chin tuck. Practice these engagements separately, then combine them.

2. Cat-Cow

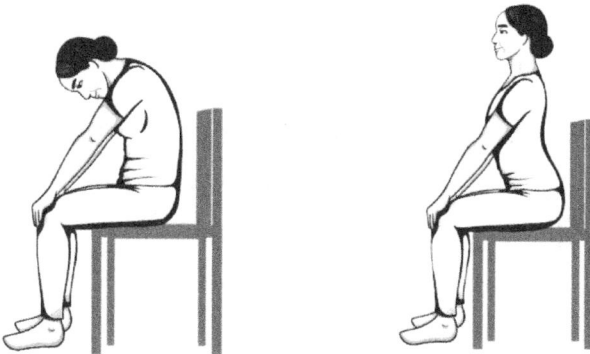

Purpose: Mobilizes the spine, promoting flexibility and improving ease of movement for bending, standing, and walking.

Instructions: Exhale as you round your back and tuck your chin (Cat). Inhale as you arch your back and look forward or slightly upward (Cow). Move slowly and repeat.

3. Forward Bend (Variation 1)

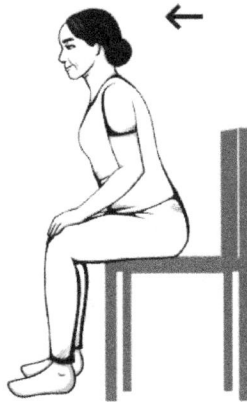

Purpose: Stretches the lower back and hamstrings, improving flexibility and balance.

Instructions: Gently hinge forward at the hips, resting your hands on your thighs or shins. Keep your back long and your head relaxed.

4. Twist (Variation 1)

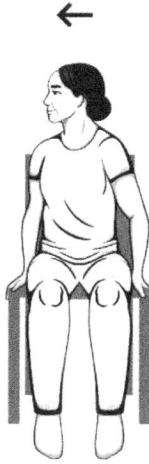

Purpose: Improves spinal rotation and back flexibility. Enhances the ability to look or reach behind and improves balance.

Instructions: Sit tall with your hands to your sides. Gently twist your torso and turn your head. Hold, then switch sides.

5. Head Turns

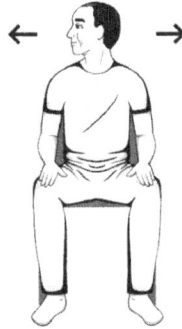

Purpose: Stretches the neck muscles, improving posture and making it easier to look behind.

Instructions: Sit tall and turn your head to one side. Hold, then switch sides.

6. Head Tilts

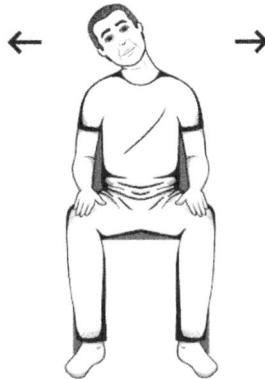

Purpose: Stretches the side neck muscles, reducing tension and supporting good posture.

Instructions: Sit tall and tilt your head to one side, bringing your ear toward your shoulder. Hold, then switch sides.

7. Head Nods

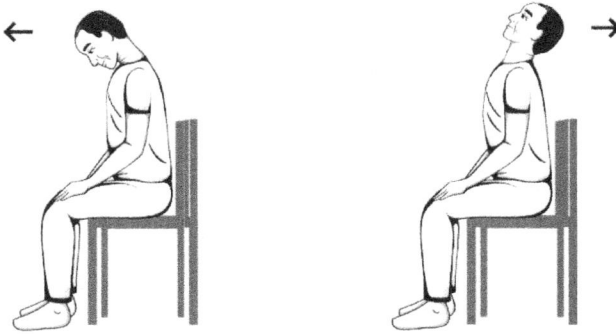

Purpose: Stretches the front and back neck muscles.

Instructions: Sit tall and slowly nod your head downward. Hold, then gently tilt your head upward.

8. Back Squeezes

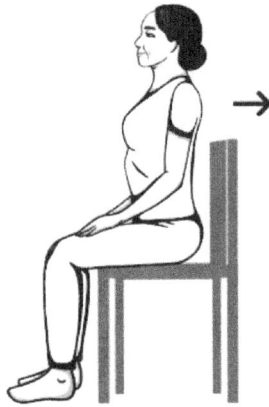

Purpose: Improves upper body posture, supporting the neck and shoulders.

Instructions: Sit tall with relaxed shoulders. Squeeze your shoulder blades together while slightly lifting your chest.

9. Shoulder Rolls

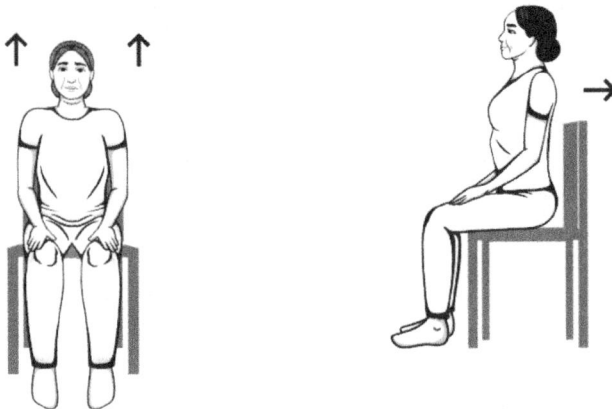

Purpose: Increases shoulder mobility, relieves tension, and supports proper posture.

Instructions: Move your shoulders backward in a circular motion, starting from a lift to a back and down motion, completing a full backward circle.

10. Forward Reach

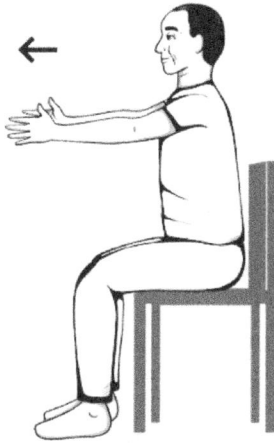

Purpose: Enhances upper body strength and postural stability.

Instructions: Sit tall, engage your core, then raise your arms forward to shoulder height.

11. Backward Reach

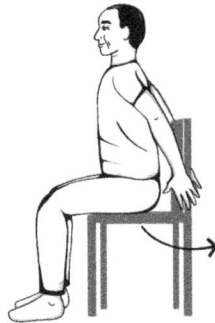

Purpose: Improves posture, opens the chest, and restores shoulder mobility.

Instructions: Reach both arms backward behind you, squeezing shoulder blades together.

12. Knee Raises

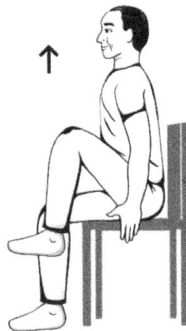

Purpose: Strengthens core stability and hip flexors, essential for standing, walking, and climbing stairs.

Instructions: Sit tall, engage your posture and core muscles, and raise one knee upward. Hold, then switch sides.

13. Knee Extensions

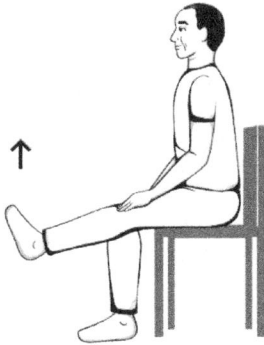

Purpose: Strengthens the quadriceps and improves knee stability, supporting standing and walking.

Instructions: Sit tall and engage your posture and core muscles. Extend one leg forward, straightening the knee. Hold, then switch sides.

14. Knee to Chest

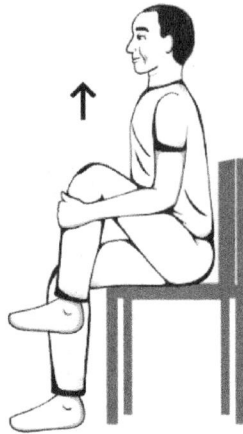

Purpose: Stretch hip and low back muscles

Instructions: Lift up a knee and use both hands to pull it toward your chest. Hold, then switch sides.

15. Figure Four

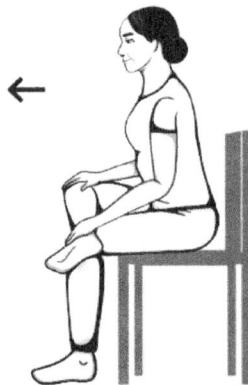

Purpose: Relieves hip and lower back tension, enhancing flexibility and upright posture.

Instructions: Cross one ankle over the opposite knee. Gently press the raised knee toward the floor.

16. Knee to Opposite Shoulder

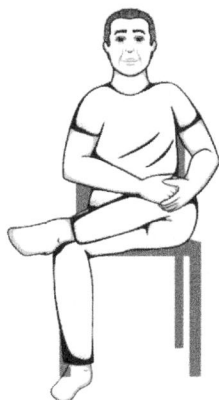

Purpose: Relieves hip and lower back tension, enhancing flexibility and mobility.

Instructions: With hands around the knee, pull the knee toward the opposite shoulder. Hold, then switch sides.

17. Hamstring Stretch with Strap

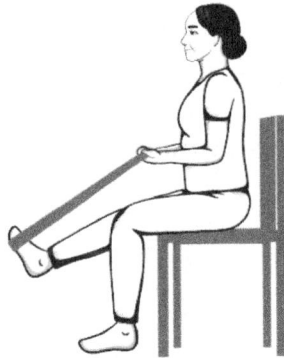

Purpose: Enhances hamstring flexibility, improving bending, balance, and walking.

Instructions: Loop a strap around one foot. Straighten the knee and gently pull the leg upward. Hold, then switch sides.

18. Lateral Side Step

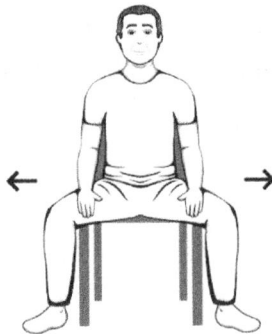

Purpose: Improves hip mobility and reduces stiffness, supporting balance and lateral movements.

Instructions: Sit tall and move one foot outward to the side, gently opening the legs. Then, move the other foot outward. You can do one leg at a time if this is uncomfortable.

"Life is like riding a bicycle. To keep your balance, you must keep moving."

— ALBERT EINSTEIN

SECTION 2: INTERMEDIATE POSES

These poses add gentle challenges to build strength and coordination. Practice these after mastering the foundational poses. Be sure to engage your pelvic, core, and postural muscles with all assertive poses for best control and safety.

1. Forward Bend (Variation 2)

Purpose: Deepens lower back and hamstring flexibility.

Instructions: Sit tall, hinge forward at the hips, and reach toward your ankles or yoga

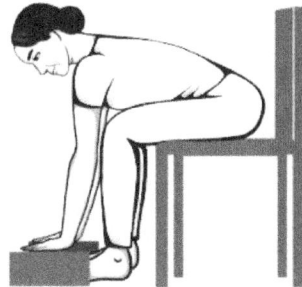

blocks. Hold while keeping your back straight.

2. Twist (Variation 2)

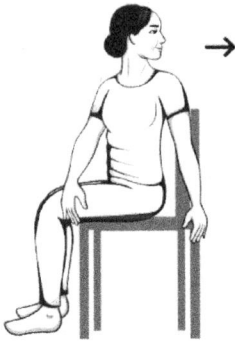

Purpose: Improves spinal rotation and stretches the back. Supports activities such as looking or reaching behind, changing directions while walking, and improving balance.

Instructions: Sit tall with your spine elongated. Place one hand on the opposite leg and the other on the side of the chair. Gently twist your torso, turning your head to follow the movement. Hold, then switch sides.

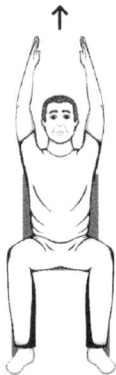

3. Overhead Reach

Purpose: Improves shoulder mobility and postural strength.

Instructions: Raise both arms overhead.

4. Lateral Reach

Purpose: Improves shoulder and postural strength.

Instructions: Extend arms out to the sides to shoulder height.

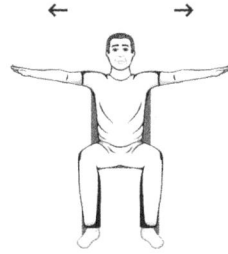

5. Pigeon Pose with Overhead Reach

Purpose: Enhances flexibility in the hips, sides of the torso, and shoulders. Straightens and lengthens the spine.

Instructions: Cross one ankle over the opposite thigh. Raise your arms overhead and hinge forward slightly.

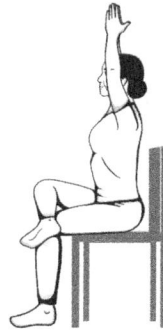

6. Side Stretch

Purpose: Stretches the sides of the torso and improves spinal mobility.

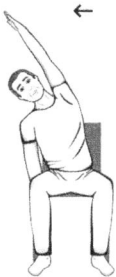

Instructions: Extend one arm overhead, reaching through your fingertips. Lean gently to the opposite side, keeping your hips grounded. Hold, then switch sides.

. . .

7. Sun Salutation Sequence (Variation 1)

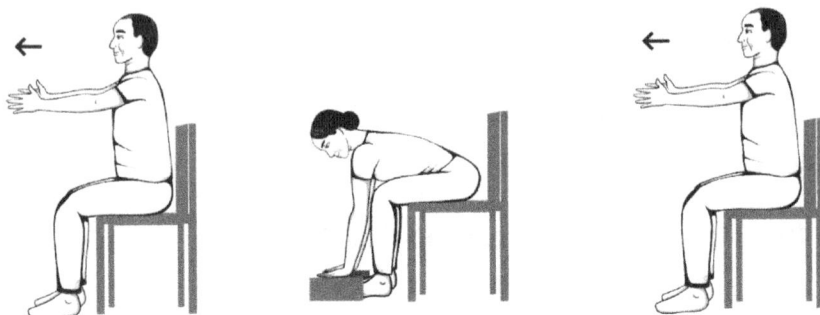

Purpose: Improves flexibility, mobility, and energy through a series of flowing movements.

Instructions:

1. Sit tall with your feet flat on the floor.
2. Inhale and raise your arms to shoulder level.
3. Exhale and fold forward, bringing your hands toward your ankles or yoga blocks.
4. Inhale and return to the upright seated position, raising your arms again.
5. Repeat this sequence 3-5 times.

These intermediate poses build upon your foundational skills, allowing you to continue strengthening your body and improving your mobility. Focus on controlled movements, steady breathing, and mindful engagement of your core and posture.

"We have a brain for one reason and one reason only — and that's to produce adaptable and complex movements."

— DANIEL WOLPERT

SECTION 3: ADVANCED POSES

These poses significantly challenge your strength, balance, and flexibility. After mastering the intermediate poses, attempt these when you feel ready and confident. The goal is to hold each pose for 3 to 5 breaths. However, build yourself up to this level as needed. As always, engage your pelvic, core, and postural muscles for the best results in all assertive poses.

1. Forward Bend (Variation 3)

Purpose: Deepens the stretch in the lower back and hamstrings, improving flexibility and balance.

Instructions: Sit tall with your feet flat on the floor. Exhale as you hinge forward at the hips, maintaining a long, straight back. Reach toward your ankles or the floor, allowing your head and neck to relax. Avoid

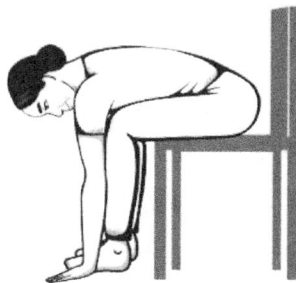

→

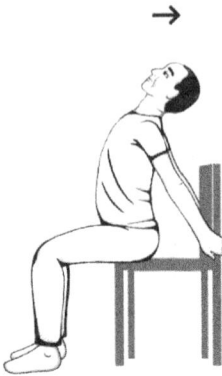

rounding your back. Hold, then return to an upright position.

2. Chest Opener

Purpose: Opens the chest and strengthens the upper back, promoting better posture.

Instructions: Place your hands on the back of the chair. Draw your shoulders back and lift your chest upward, creating a gentle arch in your upper back.

3. Supported Eagle Pose

Purpose: Stretches the shoulders, upper back, and hips while enhancing focus, balance, and posture.

Instructions:

- Sit tall with your feet flat on the floor.
- Cross one leg over the other, wrapping your foot around the planted lower leg if possible.
- Extend your arms forward and cross one arm over the other at the elbows.
- Bend your elbows and bring your palms or the backs of your hands together in front of you.

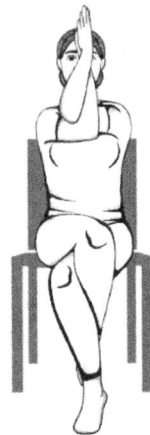

- If comfortable, lift the elbows and move the hands slightly forward.
- Hold, then switch sides.

4. Alternating Arm & Knee Raise

Purpose: Strengthens the shoulders, core, and hips, enhancing balance and coordination.

Instructions: Sit tall and engage your pelvic, core, and postural muscles. Raise one knee and the opposite arm simultaneously. Hold, then switch sides.

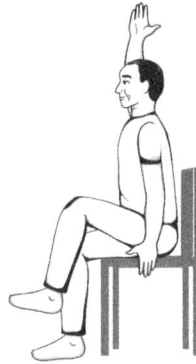

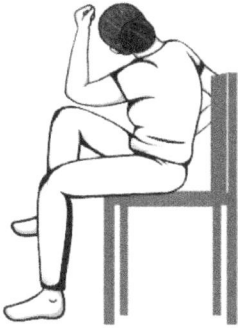

5. Elbow to Knee Twist

Purpose: Strengthens the core, trunk rotators, and hip muscles, improving coordination for activities like reaching and twisting.

Instructions: Engage your core. Lift one knee and touch it with the opposite elbow, twisting through the torso. Hold, then switch sides.

6. Supported Chair Pose

Purpose: Builds lower body, core, and back strength while improving posture and stability. This pose prepares you for standing balance and functional movements like transitioning out of a chair.

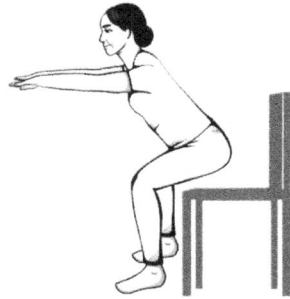

Instructions:

1. Sit at the edge of a sturdy chair with your feet hip-width apart.
2. Place your hands on your thighs or extend them forward for balance.
3. Engage your core and keep your back straight.
4. Shift your weight forward onto your feet.
5. Press your feet into the floor to activate your leg muscles and lift your hips up off the chair.
6. Hold, then repeat.

7. Sun Salutation Sequence (Variation 2)

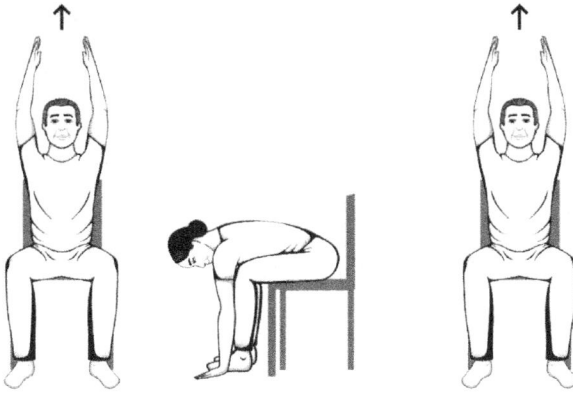

Purpose: This flowing sequence boosts circulation, flexibility, and energy.

Instructions:

1. Sit tall with your feet flat on the floor.
2. Inhale and raise your arms overhead, stretching through your spine.
3. Exhale and fold forward, bringing your hands toward your feet or the floor.
4. Inhale and return to the seated upright position, raising your arms again.
5. Repeat the sequence 3-5 times.

HOW TO USE THIS LIBRARY

Take your time exploring each pose. Start with foundational poses and progress through the intermediate and advanced variations as you build strength, flexibility, and confidence. Always listen to your body—yoga is a journey of self-discovery, not a race.

8

10-MINUTE ROUTINES FOR BEGINNERS

"Strength doesn't come from what you can do. It comes from overcoming the things you once thought you couldn't."

— RIKKI ROGERS

Welcome to your beginner routines! These sequences gently ease you into chair yoga, helping you build strength, improve flexibility, and enhance your posture and balance. Each routine can be completed in just 10 minutes, making it easy to incorporate into your daily schedule. Remember to move mindfully, take intentional breaths, and enjoy the process.

Note: A **1-breath hold** (one full inhale and exhale) equals about five seconds. If holding a pose longer than one breath is too difficult, start with what you are comfortable with. If doing two or more repetitions of a pose is too challenging, then start with one repetition. Build yourself to tolerate the longer holds and the greater repetitions as your body adapts and conditions.

Each of the four illustrated routines targets specific areas of fitness: core and trunk stability, flexibility, balance, and strength. Each 10-minute session includes a warm-up, core poses, and a cooldown to ensure a well-rounded practice.

Starting Point: Start with a **1-breath hold** and perform **1 to 3 repetitions each**.

Goal: Build yourself up to do **2 to 3 breath holds** and perform **3 to 5 repetitions each**.

ROUTINE 1: CORE STABILITY AND ALIGNMENT

Purpose: Build pelvic floor, core, and postural strength to support stability and alignment.

Warm-Ups:

- **Cat-Cow:** Exhale as you round your back and tuck your chin (Cat). Inhale as you arch your back and look straight or slightly upward (Cow).

- **Head Turns:** Rotate your head to one side and then the other.
- **Head Nods:** Move your head downward and then upward.

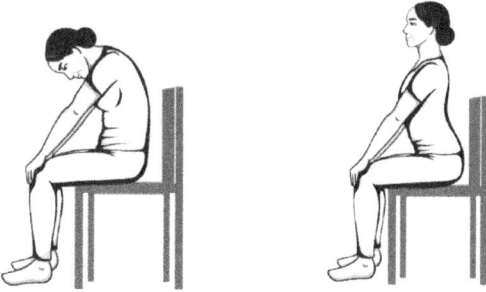

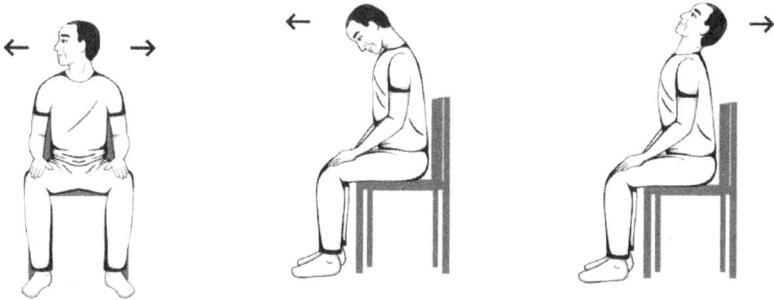

Main Poses:

- **Mountain Pose - Kegel:** Engage your pelvic floor muscles.

- **Mountain Pose - Core Engagement:** Engage your deep abdominal core muscles.
- **Mountain Pose - Back Squeezes:** Pinch your shoulder blades together.
- **Mountain Pose - Chin Tuck:** Move your head back and tuck your chin slightly down.

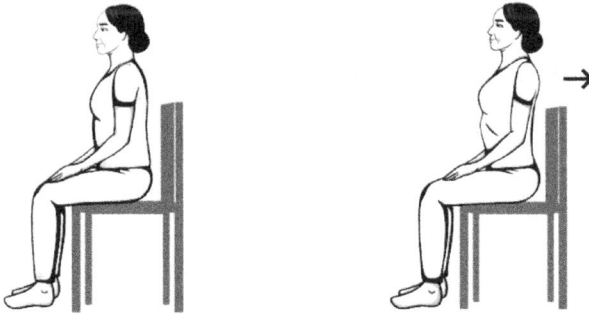

Cool-Downs:

- **Forward Bend (Variation 1):** Hinge at the hips and bend forward, resting your hands on your thighs or shins.
- **Twist (Variation 1):** Place your hands to your sides and gently twist through your torso and neck. Hold, then switch sides.

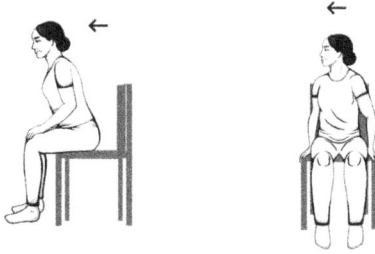

ROUTINE 2: FLEXIBILITY FOCUS

Purpose: Improve range of motion in the spine, hips, and shoulders while encouraging relaxation.

Warm-Ups:

- **Shoulder Rolls:** Roll your shoulders backward, moving them up, back, then down in a full circle.
- **Twist (Variation 1):** Twist gently to one side, keeping your hands to your sides. Hold, then switch sides.

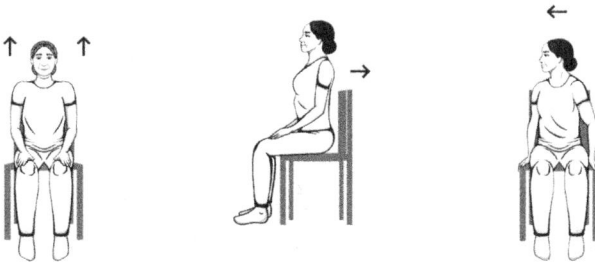

Main Poses:

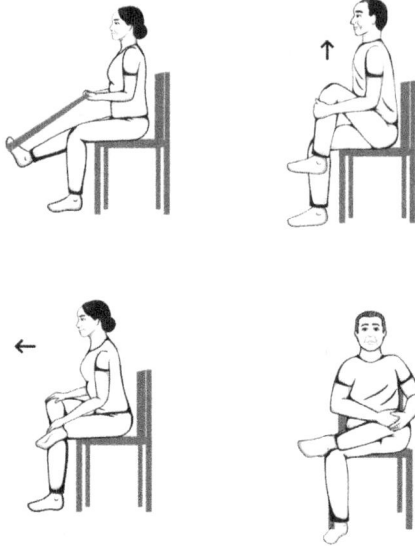

- **Hamstring Stretch with Strap:** Extend one leg forward and use a strap or towel to stretch gently. Hold, then switch sides.
- **Knee to Chest:** Lift one knee toward your chest using both hands. Hold, then switch sides.
- **Figure Four:** Cross one ankle over the opposite knee and gently press the raised knee down. Hold, then switch sides.
- **Knee to Opposite Shoulder:** Cross one ankle over the opposite knee. Use your hands to pull the knee toward the opposite shoulder. Hold, then switch sides.

Cool-Downs:

- **Forward Bend (Variation 1):** Fold gently forward, resting your hands on your thighs or shins.
- **Lateral Side Step:** Lift and move one foot outward to the side as wide as you can tolerate, planting it on the floor. Then, do the same with the other foot. Hold, bring both feet back to the center, then repeat.

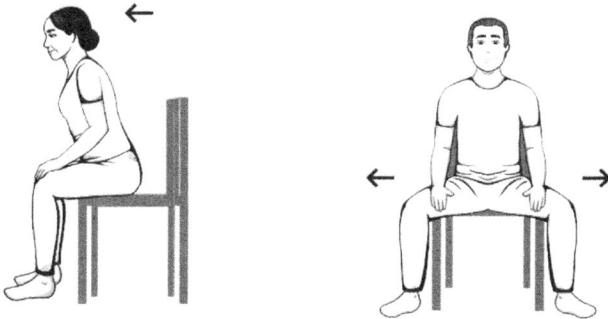

ROUTINE 3: BALANCE BASICS

Purpose: Enhance body awareness, stability, and coordination.

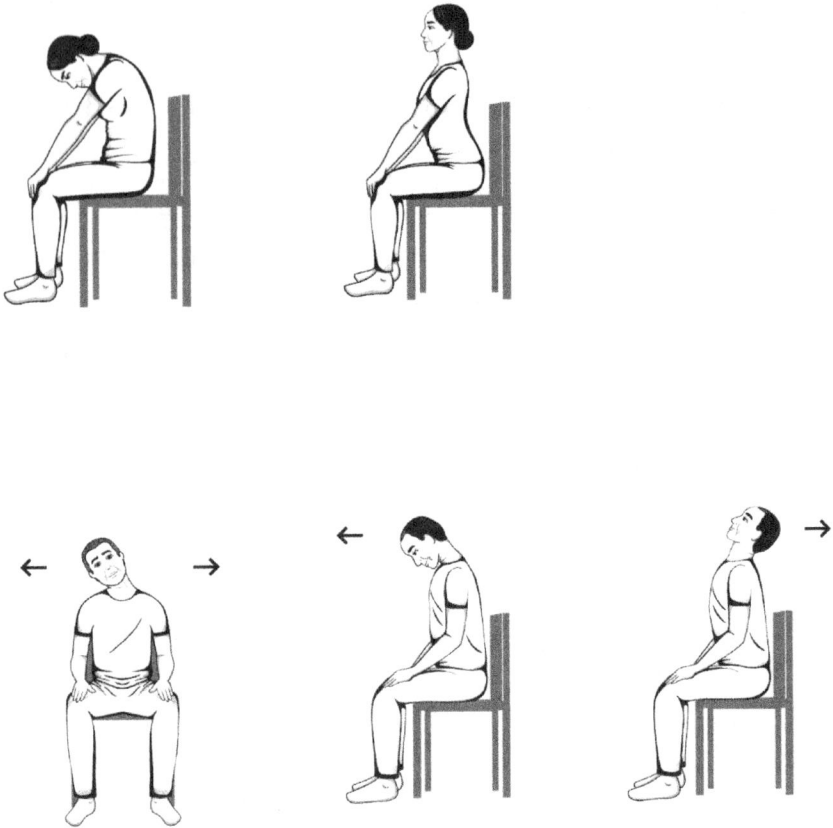

Warm-Ups:

- **Cat-Cow:** Exhale as you round your back and tuck your chin (Cat). Inhale as you arch your back and look straight or slightly upward (Cow).
- **Head Tilts:** Tilt your head laterally, moving your ear toward your shoulder. Hold, then switch sides.
- **Head Nods:** Look down and hold, then look up and hold.

Main Poses:

- **Knee Raises:** Lift one knee at a time. Hold, then switch sides.
- **Knee Extensions:** Extend one leg forward. Hold, then switch sides.
- **Lateral Side Step:** Lift and move one foot outward to the side as wide as you can tolerate, planting it on the floor. Then, do the same with the other foot. Hold, bring both feet back to the center, then repeat.

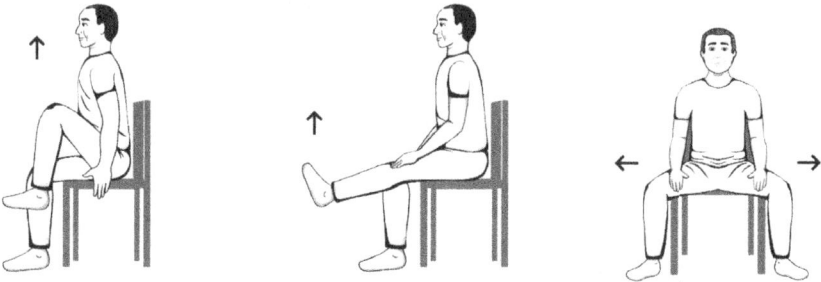

Cool-Downs:

- **Twist (Variation 1):** Twist gently to one side. Hold, then switch sides.
- **Shoulder Rolls:** Roll your shoulders backward, moving them up, back, then down in a full circle.

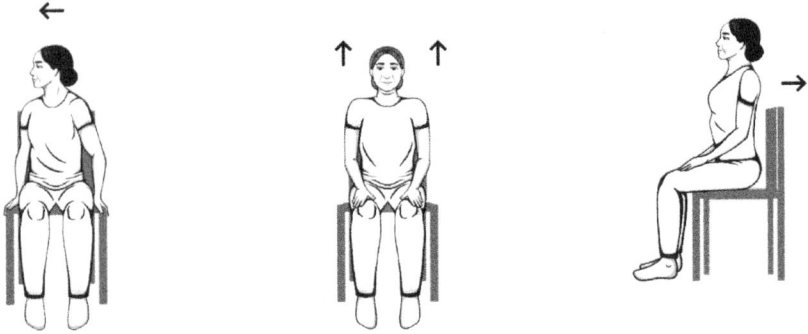

ROUTINE 4: STRENGTH BUILDER

Purpose: Strengthen key muscle groups to improve function and reduce fall risk.

Warm-Ups:

- **Cat-Cow:** Exhale as you round your back and tuck your chin (Cat). Inhale as you arch your back and look slightly upward (Cow).
- **Shoulder Rolls:** Roll your shoulders backward, moving them up, back, then down in a full circle.

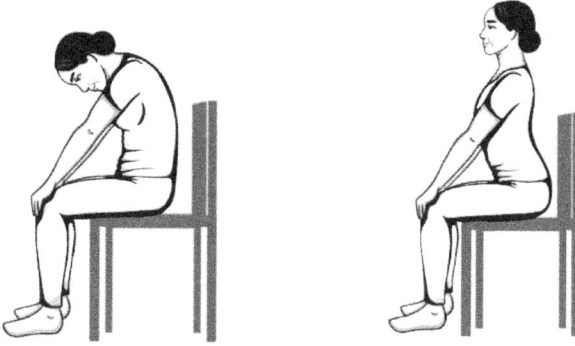

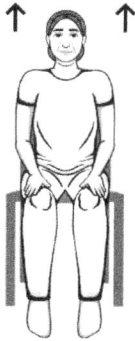

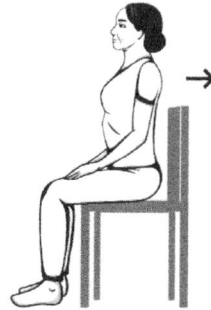

Main Poses:

- **Knee Extensions:** Straighten one leg, hold, then
  lower slowly and switch sides.
- **Lateral Reach:** Raise both arms out to the sides at
  shoulder height and hold.

- **Forward Reach:** Raise both arms forward at shoulder height and hold.
- **Backward Reach:** Reach behind through extended fingers, opening and lifting the chest forward and hold.

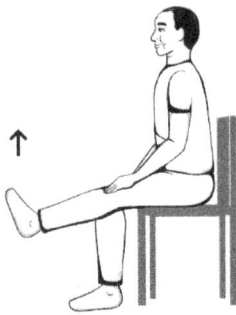

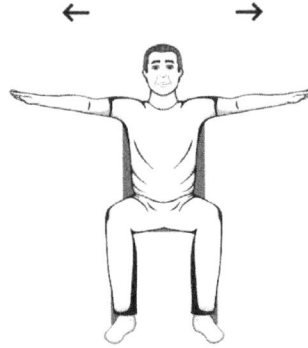

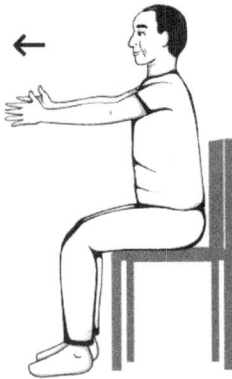

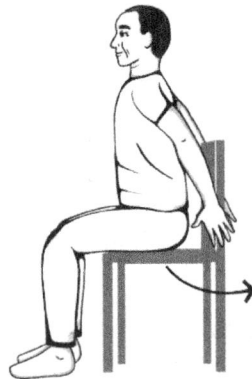

Cool-Downs:

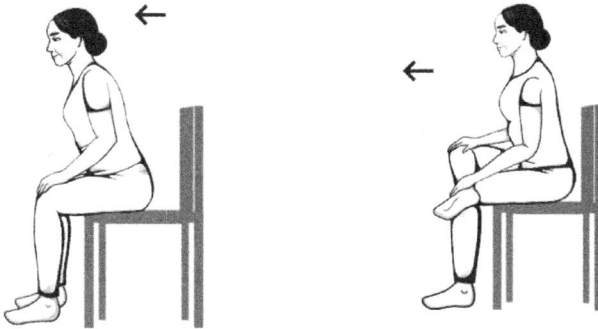

- **Forward Bend (Variation 1):** Fold gently forward with your hands resting on your thighs or shins.
- **Figure Four:** Cross one ankle over the opposite knee and gently press the crossed knee down. Hold, then switch sides.

Closing Notes

Congratulations on completing these beginner routines! Consistency is key. With regular practice, you'll notice improvements in your strength, flexibility, and overall well-being.

A recommendation: Select one of the four routines to practice daily for a week, and then move on to do the same with the others. You can then establish a weekly plan of rotating through the four routines every four days. As you grow more comfortable, you can explore intermediate and advanced routines in the following chapters. Always listen to your body, and remember that progress is a journey.

SHARE YOUR THOUGHTS!

By now, you've learned how the body ages with time and how **tailored chair yoga** can progressively impact positive physical and mental change. Before moving forward to the next chapter, I have a small but **important request**—take just a few minutes now to leave an Amazon Review.

Your feedback helps others discover this resource and ensures it reaches those most need it. **Your review makes a difference!**

Thank you for being part of this movement to bring **safe, effective, and empowering** resources like this guide to seniors and their families.

Go to this link:
https://a.co/d/ggZBQ6S
Or scan this QR code with your phone camera:

1. Click on the **review ratings** and select the "**Write a Review**" button.
2. Share just a few sentences about the part of the book that you liked the most so far.
3. Take a picture of your favorite page, quote, or book cover, and upload it to your review.
4. Title your review.
5. Press the yellow "**Submit**" button.

With gratitude,
Movement Freedom Publications

9

10-MINUTE ROUTINES FOR INTERMEDIATES

"Success is the sum of small efforts repeated day in and day out."

— ROBERT COLLIER

B y now, you have mastered the routines at the beginner level and feel able to progress to the next level. With that said, congratulations! You have reached the intermediate level of your chair yoga journey! Your dedication and consistency have brought you here, and that's something to celebrate. With your newfound strength and confidence, these intermediate routines are a progression designed to help you build upon the foundation you've already established. Remember, yoga is a personal practice—always listen to your body, engage your core and postural muscles with every assertive pose, and avoid any movement that causes discomfort or pain. It's perfectly fine to revisit the beginner routines if new ones are too challenging—progress at your own pace.

Each routine continues to focus on these areas: core and trunk stability, flexibility, balance, and strength. Every 10-minute session includes a warm-up, core poses, and a cooldown to provide a well-rounded practice.

Starting Point: Start with **1 to 2 breath holds** and perform **2 to 3 repetitions each**.

Goal: Build yourself up to do **2 to 3 breath holds** and perform **3 to 5 repetitions each**.

ROUTINE 1: CORE AND TRUNK STABILITY

Purpose: Build pelvic floor, core, and postural strength to support spinal stability and alignment.

Warm-Up:

- **Cat-Cow:** Exhale as you round your back and tuck your chin (Cat). Inhale as you arch your back and look straight or slightly upward (Cow).
- **Head Turns:** Rotate your head to one side. Hold, then switch sides.

- **Head Nods:** Move your head downward and hold.
  Then, move your head upward and hold.

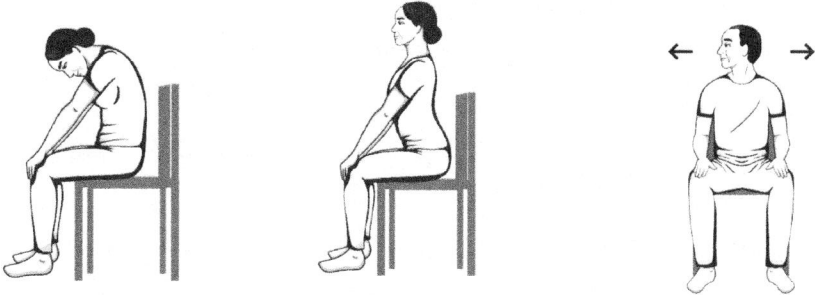

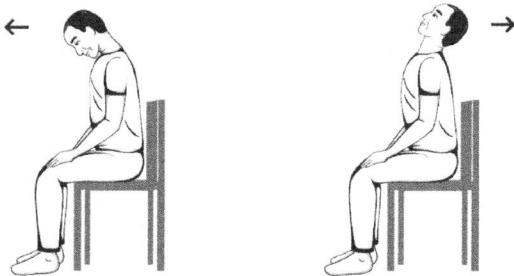

Core Poses:

- **Mountain Pose – Core and Pelvic Engagement:**
  Engage your pelvic floor muscles while drawing
  your lower abdomen inward and upward toward
  your spine. Hold, maintaining a relaxed upper body.
- **Mountain Pose – Core and Upper Body
  Engagement:** Engage your deep abdominal core

muscles by drawing your lower abdomen inward and upward toward your spine. At the same time, gently pinch your shoulder blades together, keeping your shoulders relaxed and down.

- **Overhead Reach with Upper Body Engagement:** Raise both arms overhead while keeping your shoulders relaxed. Gently tuck your chin and engage your shoulder blades.
- **Knee Raises:** Engage the core, then lift one knee and hold. Then, switch sides.

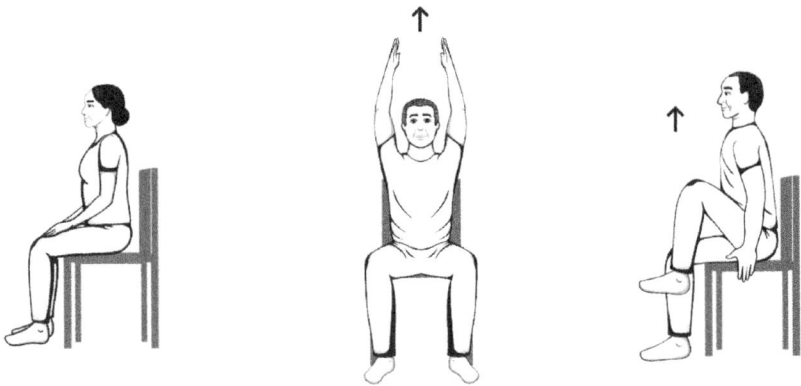

Cooldown:

- **Forward Bend (Variation 2):** Sit at the edge of your chair and hinge forward at the hips, reaching for your ankles or yoga blocks.
- **Side Stretch:** Sit tall and reach your right arm

overhead, leaning gently to the left. Hold, then switch sides.

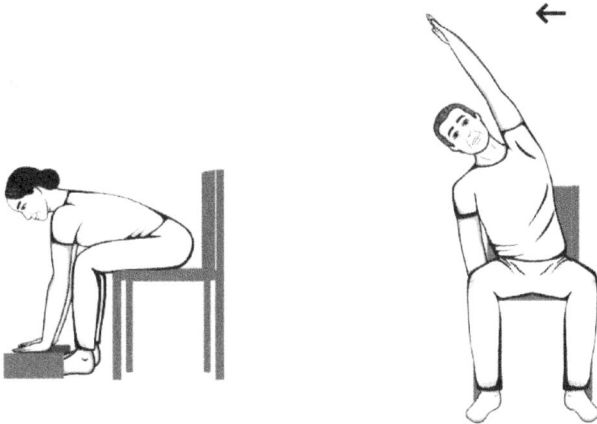

ROUTINE 2: FLEXIBILITY FOCUS

Purpose: Improve range of motion in the spine, hips, and shoulders while encouraging relaxation.

Warm-Up:

- **Cat-Cow:** Exhale as you round your back and tuck your chin (Cat). Inhale as you arch your back and look straight or slightly upward (Cow).
- **Head Tilts:** Slowly tilt your head to the right, bringing your ear toward your shoulder. Hold, then repeat on the left.
- **Head Nods:** Move your head downward and hold. Then look up and hold.

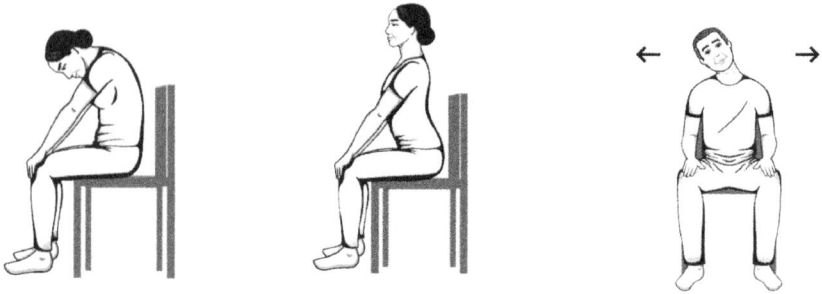

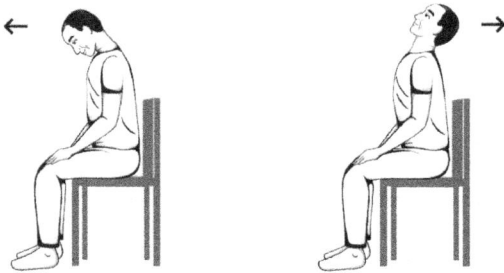

Core Poses:

- **Hamstring Stretch with Strap:** Sit tall and extend your right leg forward with your heel resting on the floor. Loop a strap or towel around the ball of your foot and gently lift your foot off the floor to stretch your hamstring. Hold, then switch legs.
- **Side Stretch:** Sit tall and reach your right arm overhead, leaning gently to the left. Hold, then switch sides.

- **Seated Twist (Variation 2):** Place your left hand on your opposite thigh. Turn your body to the right, placing your right hand on the backrest. Gently twist your torso and turn your head to follow. Hold, then switch sides.
- **Pigeon Pose with Overhead Reach:** Sit slightly forward in your chair. Place your right ankle on your left thigh. Raise your hands overhead and clasp them together. Hold, then switch sides.

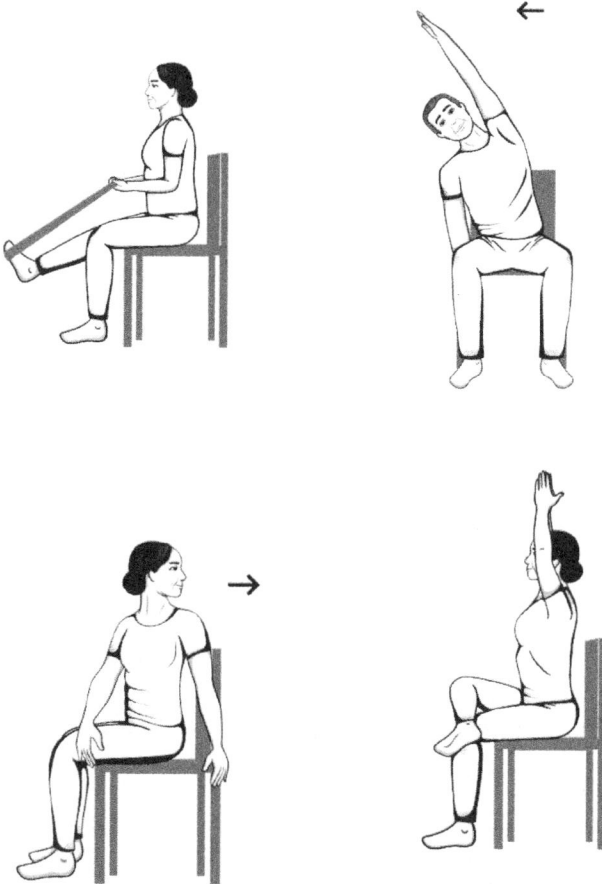

Cooldown:

- **Forward Bend (Variation 2):** Sit at the edge of your chair and hinge forward at the hips, reaching for your ankles or yoga blocks.
- **Shoulder Rolls:** Sit tall and roll your shoulders backward slowly, starting with a lift, then moving them back and down into a full circle.

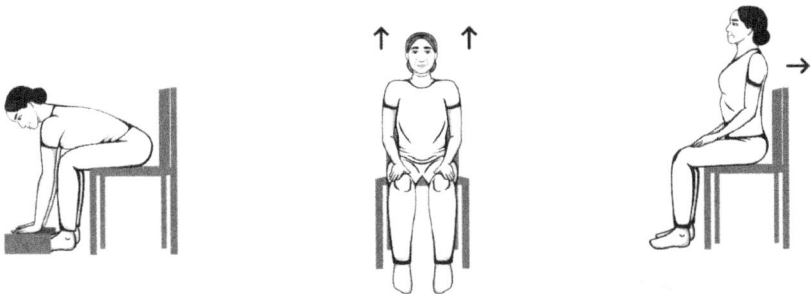

ROUTINE 3: BALANCE BASICS

Purpose: Enhance body awareness, stability, and coordination.

Warm-Up:

- **Back Squeezes:** Sit tall and gently pinch your shoulder blades together, keeping your shoulders relaxed and down.
- **Side Stretch:** Sit tall and reach your right arm

overhead, leaning gently to the left. Hold, then switch sides.

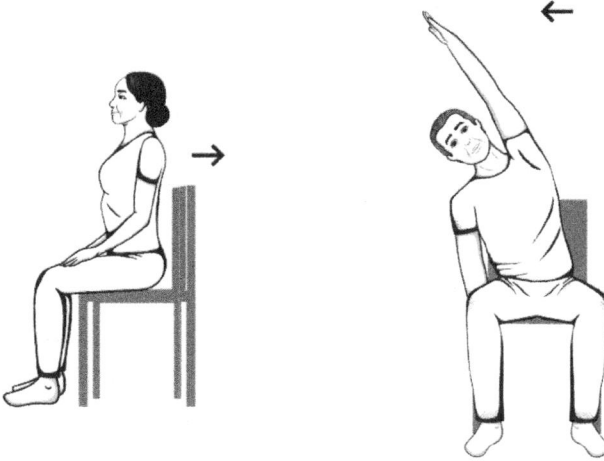

Core Poses:

- **Sun Salutation Sequence (Variation 1):** Begin in seated mountain pose. Inhale and raise your arms forward to shoulder height. Exhale and hinge forward into a seated forward bend, reaching for ankles or yoga blocks. Inhale to return to mountain pose with arms raised.
- **Alternating Arm and Leg Raises:** Sit tall and engage your core. Extend your right arm overhead while lifting your left leg. Hold, then switch sides.
- **Chest Opener:** Sit tall and place your hands on the chair's backrest. Gently press your chest forward and lift your gaze, creating a slight arch in your back.

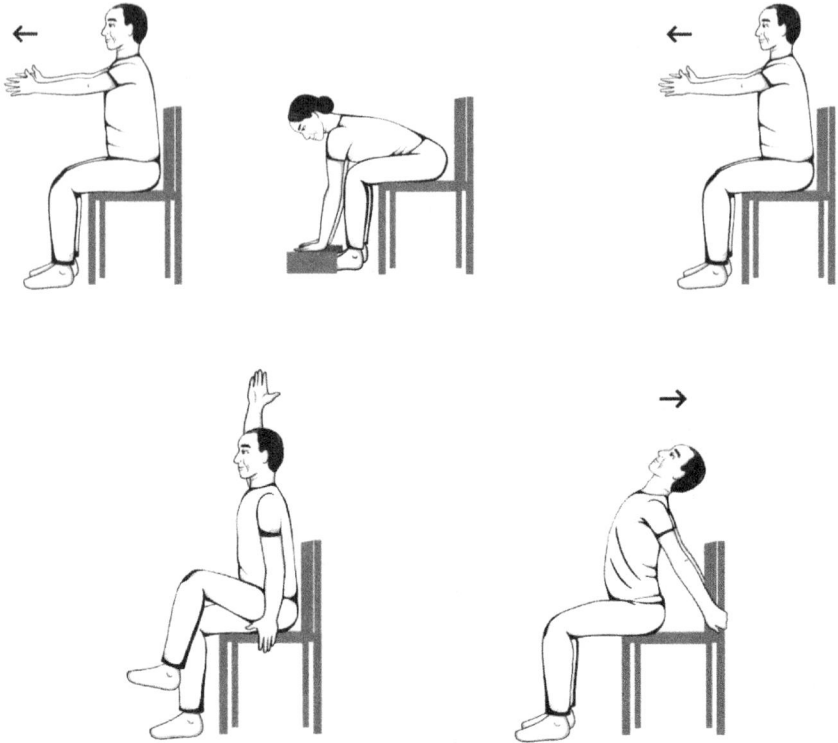

Cooldown:

- **Seated Twist (Variation 2):** Place your left hand on your opposite thigh. Turn your body to the right, placing your right hand on the backrest. Gently twist your torso and turn your head to follow. Hold, then switch sides.
- **Lateral Side Step:** Lift and move one foot outward to the side as wide as you can tolerate, planting it on the floor. Then, do the same with the other foot. Hold, bring both feet back to the center, then repeat.

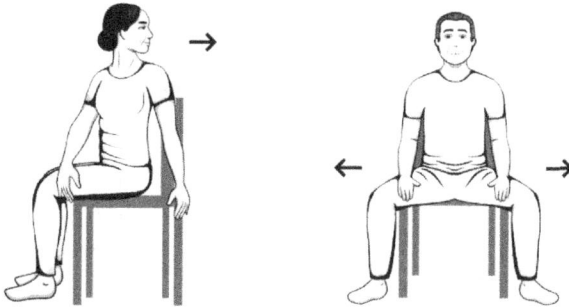

ROUTINE 4: STRENGTH BUILDER

Purpose: Strengthen key muscle groups to improve function and reduce fall risk.

Warm-Up:

- **Seated Twist (Variation 2):** Place your left hand on your opposite thigh. Turn your body to the right, placing your right hand on the backrest. Gently twist your torso and turn your head to follow. Hold, then switch sides.
- **Forward Bend (Variation 2):** Sit at the edge of your chair and hinge forward at the hips, reaching for your ankles or yoga blocks.

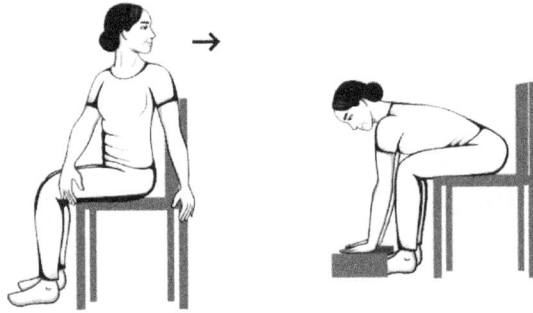

Core Poses:

- **Pigeon Pose with Overhead Reach:** Sit slightly forward in your chair. Place your right ankle on your left thigh. Raise your hands overhead and clasp them together. Hold, then switch sides.
- **Lateral Reach:** Extend your arms out to the sides at shoulder height. Engage your core and scapular muscles to support the movement, hold and lower arms down, and then repeat.
- **Backward Reach:** Move your hands behind you, extending your shoulders and keeping your back straight. Engage your core, scapular muscles, and chin tuck. Hold, relax arms, then repeat.

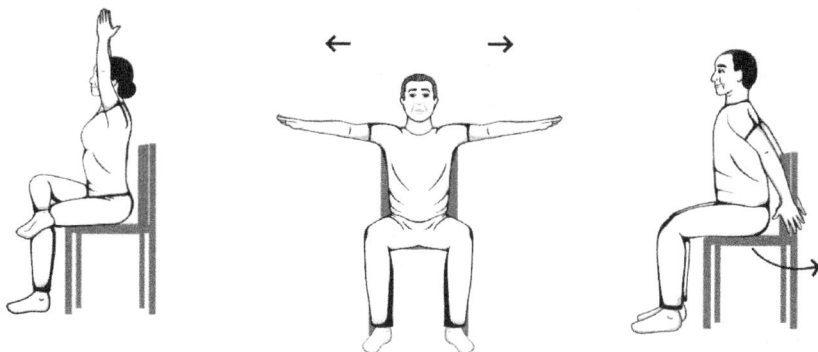

Cooldown:

- **Knee to Chest:** Lift one knee toward your chest using both hands. Hold, then switch sides.
- **Back Squeezes:** Sit tall and gently pinch your shoulder blades together, keeping your shoulders relaxed and down.

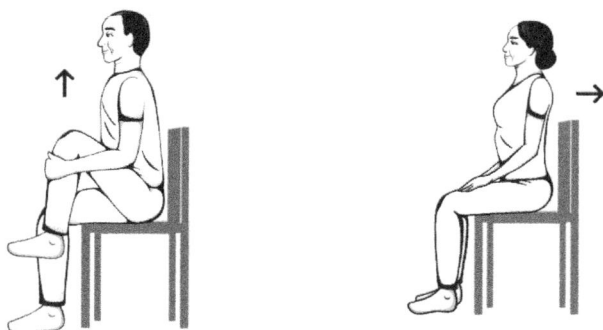

With regular practice, these intermediate routines will help you continue building strength, flexibility, and balance.

Adjust poses as needed to suit your body's unique needs and capabilities. Celebrate your progress, and prepare for more advanced challenges ahead!

A recommendation: Select one of the four routines to practice daily for a week, then do the same with the others. You can then establish a weekly plan of rotating through the four routines every four days. As you grow more comfortable, you can explore the advanced routines in the following chapter. As always, listen to your body, and remember that progress takes time and repetition.

10-MINUTE ROUTINES FOR ADVANCED LEVEL

"Progress is not achieved by luck or accident, but by working on yourself daily."

— EPICTETUS

H ats off to you for reaching the advanced level of your chair yoga practice! Your dedication, strength, and focus have brought you to this point. These advanced routines challenge your balance, flexibility, strength, and control, helping you reach new milestones.

By now, you are a master at listening to your body and progressing at your own pace. Engage your core and postural muscles with every movement, and remember that it's perfectly fine to revisit intermediate routines if needed. Your safety and comfort are essential to your success.

To recap, each 10-minute routine focuses on a specific area: core and trunk stability, enhanced flexibility, balance with movement control, and full-body strength. Each includes a warm-up, core poses, and a cooldown.

Starting Point: Start with **1 to 2 breath holds** and perform **2 to 3 repetitions each**.

Goal: Build yourself up to do **2 to 3 breath holds** and perform **3 to 5 repetitions each**.

ROUTINE 1: CORE AND TRUNK STABILITY

Warm-Up

- **Cat-Cow:** Exhale as you round your back and tuck your chin (Cat). Inhale as you arch your back and look straight or slightly upward (Cow).
- **Side Stretch:** Sit tall and reach your right arm overhead, leaning gently to the left. Hold, then switch sides.

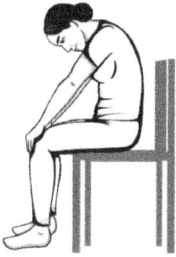

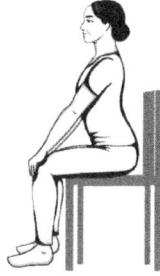

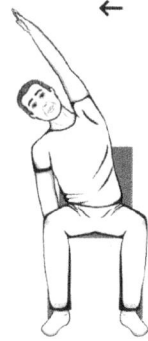

Core Poses

- **Mountain Pose with Full Pelvic and Trunk Engagement:** Sit tall and engage these trunk muscle systems in this order: first your pelvic floor, then core muscles, then scapular retractors, and finally chin tuck. Hold all simultaneously, relax, then repeat.
- **Alternating Arm and Leg Raises:** Engage your core as you simultaneously lift your right arm and left leg. Hold, switch sides, and repeat.
- **Elbow to Knee Twist:** Bring your elbow and raised opposite knee toward each other. Hold, return to the center, switch sides, and repeat.

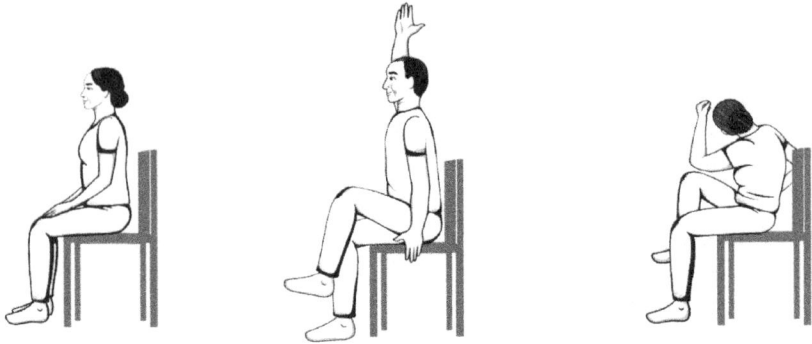

Cooldown

- **Forward Bend (Variation 3):** Sit at the edge of your chair and hinge forward at the hips, reaching for your ankles or the floor.
- **Chest Opener:** Extend your arms backward, reaching for and holding the back of the chair, arch your back gently, move your chest forward, lift your gaze, and hold.

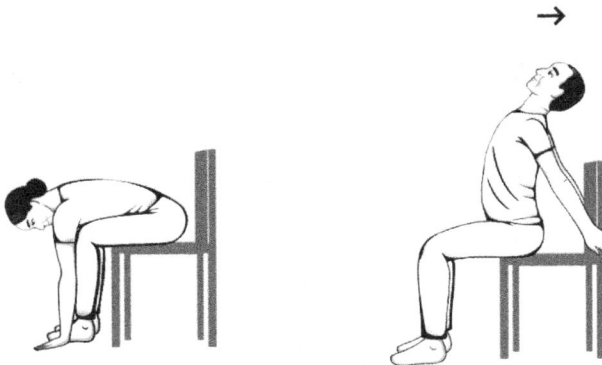

→

ROUTINE 2: ENHANCED FLEXIBILITY

Warm-Up

- **Cat-Cow Stretch:** Alternate rounding and arching your back with synchronized arm movements for deeper stretching.
- **Head Tilts:** Slowly tilt your head to the right, bringing your ear toward your shoulder. Hold, then repeat on the left.

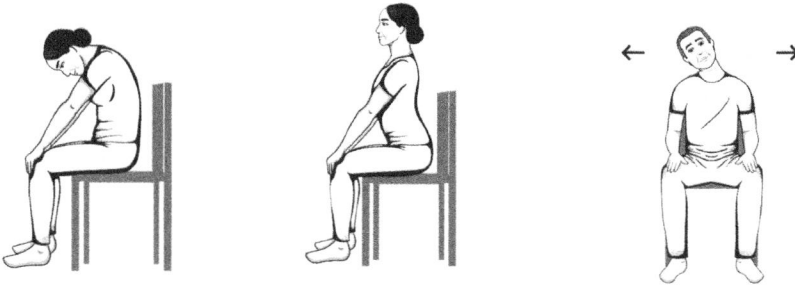

Core Poses

- **Knee to Opposite Shoulder:** Cross one ankle over the opposite knee. Use your hands to pull the knee toward the opposite shoulder. Hold, then switch sides.
- **Chest Opener:** Extend your arms backward, reaching for and holding the back of the chair, arch

your back gently, move your chest forward, and lift your gaze.

- **Pigeon Pose with Overhead Reach:** Place your ankle over the opposite thigh, raise your hands toward the ceiling, and hold. Switch sides and repeat.
- **Seated Eagle Pose:** Cross one leg over the other and wrap your arms in front, bringing the palms or backs of your hands together. Gently lift your elbows and hold. Switch sides and repeat.

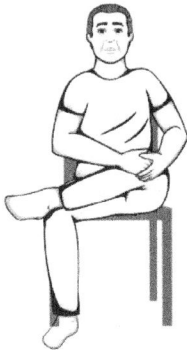

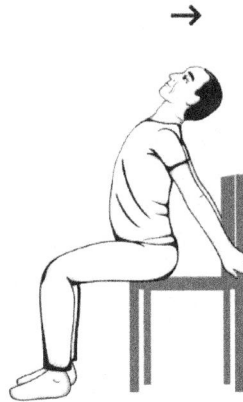

$\rightarrow$

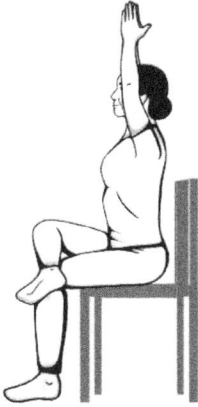

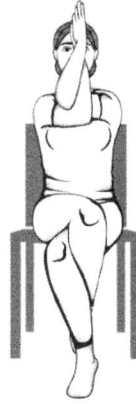

Cooldown

- **Forward Bend (Variation 3):** Sit at the edge of your chair and hinge forward at the hips, reaching for your ankles or the floor.
- **Side Stretch:** Sit tall and reach your right arm overhead, leaning gently to the left. Hold, then switch sides.

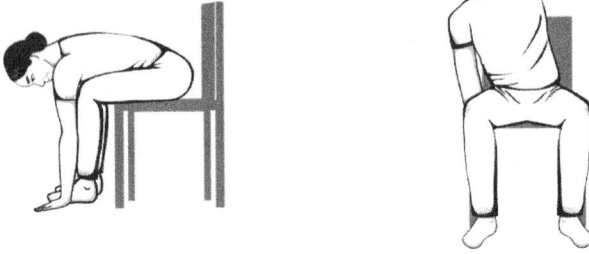

ROUTINE 3: BALANCE WITH MOVEMENT CONTROL

Warm-Up

- **Lateral Side Step:** Lift and move one foot outward to the side as wide as you can tolerate, planting it on the floor. Then, do the same with the other foot. Hold, bring both feet back to the center, then repeat.
- **Hamstring Stretch with Strap:** Sit tall and extend your right leg forward with your heel resting on the floor. Loop a strap or towel around the ball of your foot and gently lift your foot off the floor to stretch your hamstring. Hold, then switch legs.

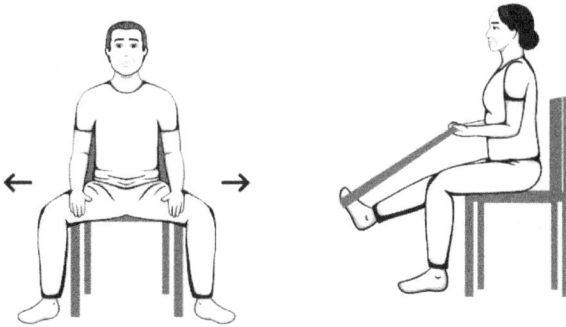

Core Poses

- **Seated Eagle Pose:** Cross one leg over the other and wrap your arms in front, bringing the palms or backs of your hands together. Gently lift your elbows and hold. Switch sides and repeat.
- **Alternating Arm and Leg Raise:** Extend your right and left leg simultaneously. Hold, switch sides, then repeat.
- **Elbow to Knee Twist:** Bring your right elbow and raised left knee toward each other. Hold, return to the center, switch sides, and repeat.
- **Supported Chair Pose:** Sit slightly forward on your chair, lift your arms to shoulder height, engage your core, transfer weight from your hips to your legs and feet, and lift your hips up off the seat. Hold and repeat.

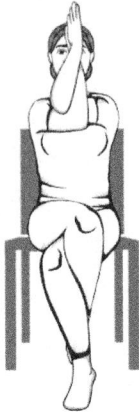

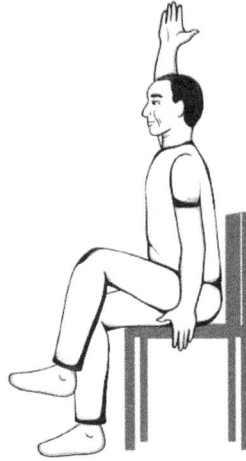

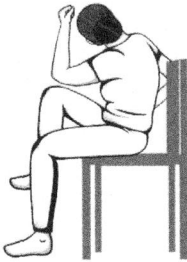

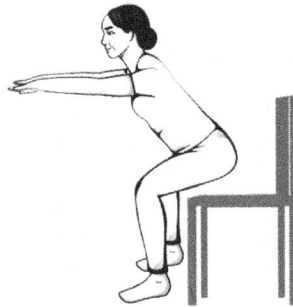

Cooldown

- **Forward Bend (Variation 3):** Sit at the edge of your chair and hinge forward at the hips, reaching for your ankles or the floor.
- **Twist (Variation 2):** Place your left hand on your opposite thigh. Turn your body to the right, placing your right hand on the backrest. Gently twist your

torso and turn your head to follow. Hold, then switch sides.

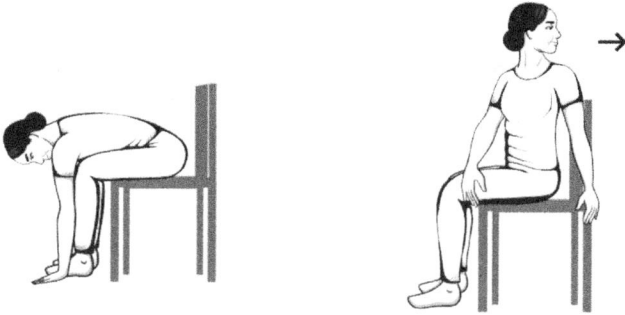

ROUTINE 4: FULL-BODY STRENGTH

Warm-Up

- **Pigeon Pose with Overhead Reach:** Place your ankle over the opposite thigh, raise your hands toward the ceiling, and hold. Switch sides and repeat.
- **Twist (Variation 2):** Place your left hand on your opposite thigh. Turn your body to the right, placing your right hand on the backrest. Gently twist your torso and turn your head to follow. Hold, then switch sides.

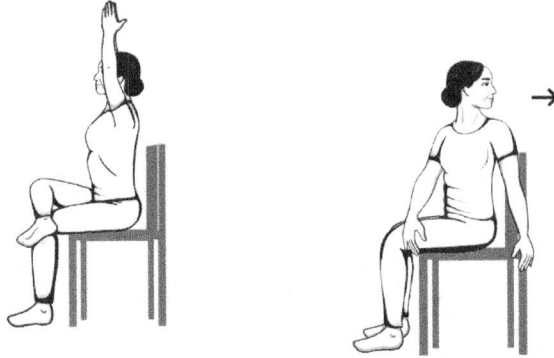

Core Poses

- **Seated Sun Salutation (Variation 2):** Flow through a sequence of overhead reach, forward fold, and seated mountain pose. Repeat.
- **Elbow to Knee Twist:** Bring your elbow toward the opposite knee and hold. Switch sides and repeat.
- **Chair Pose:** Shift your weight forward and press through your legs to lift hips up off the chair. Hold and repeat.

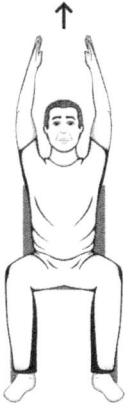

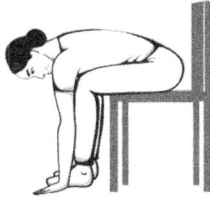

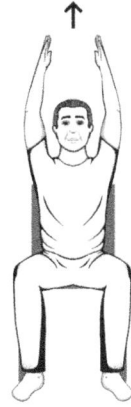

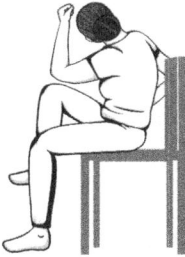

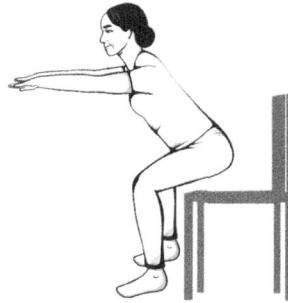

Cooldown

- **Chest Opener:** Extend your arms backward reaching for and holding the back of the chair, arch your back gently, move your chest forward, lift your gaze, and hold.
- **Forward Bend (Variation 3):** Hinge forward, reach for the floor, and hold.
- **Knee to Opposite Shoulder:** Cross one ankle over the opposite knee. Use your hands to pull the knee

toward the opposite shoulder. Hold, then switch sides.

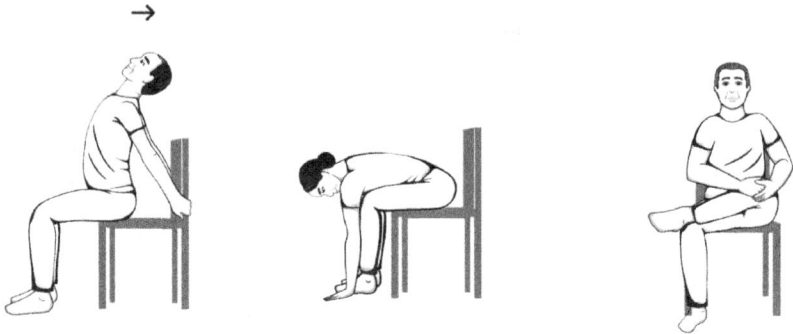

As recommended at the start of this chapter, start where you are comfortable with breath holds and repetitions, then build yourself up to the listed goal. Keep practicing and challenging yourself. Advanced routines are about refining your control, building strength, and enjoying the flow of your yoga practice! At this point, you can create your own daily and weekly routines, pulling from all the above poses. Have fun, and stay consistent!

Bonus Challenge: you can further progress your practice using a **weighted stability exercise ball** instead of a chair. I have led advanced classes incorporating a stability ball and music, and it truly elevates the practice to an even higher level. However, before advancing to this level, and for safety reasons, it's essential to have **strong balance, core stability, pelvic floor control, and postural strength**.

I initially recommend using a **stability base** under your ball for added support. Once you can confidently perform all routines across all levels, you can progress to using the ball without the base for a greater challenge.

11

INTEGRATING CHAIR YOGA INTO DAILY LIFE

"We are what we repeatedly do. Excellence, then, is not an act, but a habit."

— ARISTOTLE

I understand how challenging it can be to integrate a new exercise routine into an already full schedule. In the senior years, priorities shift—some have never-ending doctor appointments. Others have company, children, and grandchildren almost every week. Retirees have filled their schedules with weekly commitments like playing samba or mahjong every Wednesday and Friday, enjoying the must-see entertainment at the square, or playing pre-planned golf games here in The Villages. I wouldn't ask you to give up any activity that brings you joy.

Instead, I encourage you to **review your calendar** and identify a consistent time each day when you're generally free. Treat your **chair yoga practice** like any other important appointment—one that supports your strength, flexibility, and overall well-being. It's not about finding the perfect setting or the perfect time. Add your 10-minute chair yoga practice to your calendar in a way that fits your lifestyle. For best comfort, I suggest you warm up your muscles using a hot pack or heating pad on your neck and back or sit in the jacuzzi for 10 minutes before completing your 10-minute chair yoga routine. Clients tell me that heating before exercise is the best combination for comfort and participation.

Whether your goal is to **improve mobility, reduce pain, enhance relaxation, or maintain independence**, chair yoga offers a flexible, sustainable solution tailored to your needs. The key is consistency—finding a routine that works for you and making it a natural part of your day.

START WITH SELF- ASSESSMENT AND REALISTIC GOALS

Ask yourself this question: Why is it important for you to restore strength and improve movement abilities? Think about all the activities that are important in your life that you want to maintain safely and pain-free. Think about activities you have had to give up recently because of pain or difficulty. Realize that the four routines in this book on core stability, flexibility, balance, and strength are safe and effective stepping-stones that can significantly help. A **clear purpose** will guide your practice and help each session feel meaningful.

Equally important is recognizing your limitations—adapt poses to avoid discomfort or strain. Chair yoga emphasizes **progress over perfection**, allowing you to honor your body's needs. As previously recommended, all participants should start at the beginner level, which will help identify individual body needs.

BUILDING CONSISTENCY

Consistency is essential to long-term success. Choose a time that aligns with your energy levels. Morning sessions can energize you for the day, while evening practices can promote relaxation. Treat your yoga sessions as non-negotiable self-care appointments.

Life is unpredictable, so allow for flexibility. On low-energy days, focus on gentle stretches and breathing. On days when you feel more energized, challenge yourself with more advanced poses or longer breath holds. This adaptable approach makes your routine more sustainable.

TRACKING PROGRESS TO STAY MOTIVATED

Monitoring your progress can boost motivation and reinforce your commitment. Use a journal to log details such as:

- Frequency and duration of sessions
- Routines practiced
- Physical improvements (e.g., reduced stiffness, better balance)
- Emotional observations (e.g., improved mood, relaxation)

Regularly reviewing these reflections will highlight your progress and help identify areas where adjustments are needed.

OVERCOMING BARRIERS TO MOTIVATION

It's normal to experience dips in motivation. On those days, remind yourself of the benefits of a 10-minute practice—reducing stiffness, boosting energy, and improving focus. **Visualization techniques** can also help; imagine how good you'll feel after completing a session.

Introduce variety to keep your routine engaging. Rotate between different poses within a routine or different routines. Create your own routine incorporating poses from each of the four depicted categories. Play a specific song or playlist for each category or routine. Music can be motivating, so find what motivates you. Joining a class or finding an accountability partner can provide external support and encouragement.

CHAIR YOGA AS A COMPLEMENT TO PHYSICAL THERAPY

For those recovering from surgery or managing chronic conditions, chair yoga can complement physical therapy by promoting joint mobility, reducing stiffness, and enhancing circulation.

Work with your physical therapist to tailor yoga exercises to your needs. As your strength and flexibility improve, your therapist can recommend advanced modifications to keep you progressing safely.

CELEBRATING MILESTONES

Acknowledging your progress—no matter how small—is key to staying motivated. Celebrate achievements like mastering a new pose, completing a month of consistent practice, or feeling more confident in your movements. **Treat yourself to small rewards**, like new yoga props, and share your successes with friends and family.

Final Thoughts

Integrating chair yoga into your daily life will take time until it becomes a regular routine. With consistent effort, mindful tracking, and a focus on adaptability, your practice can become a cornerstone of your health and functionality. Approach each session with **patience and purpose**, and you'll experience profound improvements in both physical and mental well-being.

Remember, chair yoga isn't just exercise—it's a **lifestyle**. By embracing it fully, you invest in your health, nurture resilience, and lay the foundation for a more vibrant and active future.

12

COMMUNITY AND SUPPORT – FINDING YOUR CHAIR YOGA TRIBE

"Connection is why we're here. It's what gives purpose and meaning to our lives."

— BRENÉ BROWN

E ngaging with a community can greatly enhance your chair yoga experience. Being part of a group provides motivation, accountability, and opportunities to learn from others. Shared practice fosters consistency and personal growth while building a sense of belonging. Whether through local classes or online communities, these connections can amplify the benefits of your chair yoga journey.

FINDING LOCAL CHAIR YOGA GROUPS AND CLASSES

Community centers, senior centers, and recreation facilities often offer chair yoga classes for various experience levels. These classes provide professional guidance and a regular schedule to help you stay engaged. Group settings allow you to connect with others who share your goals, creating opportunities for new friendships and shared learning.

Workshops and special events offer additional ways to deepen your practice. These gatherings often feature guest instructors, themed sessions, or focus areas like balance or stress relief. Check community boards, libraries, or online directories to find these opportunities.

LEVERAGING ONLINE COMMUNITIES FOR SUPPORT

Online platforms offer global access to chair yoga communities. Social media groups, wellness forums, and yoga apps provide spaces to share experiences, ask questions, and access resources.

Participating in virtual communities can sustain your motivation, especially if in-person classes aren't accessible. Many groups offer live sessions, allowing you to practice with others in real time.

These online interactions can introduce new ideas and provide valuable support during challenging periods.

BUILDING YOUR OWN CHAIR YOGA COMMUNITY

If local options are limited, consider starting your own chair yoga group. Invite friends or neighbors to join regular sessions at a comfortable location, such as your home or a community room.

Platforms like Zoom or Skype make organizing group sessions easy for virtual gatherings. Whether casual or structured, these meet-ups foster accountability and camaraderie, turning chair yoga into a shared experience.

THE VALUE OF CONNECTION IN CHAIR YOGA

Community support enhances both the physical and emotional benefits of chair yoga. Shared practice encourages consistency, reduces isolation, and offers gentle accountability.

Surrounding yourself with others who share your goals reinforces the importance of self-care. Group challenges, shared milestones, and conversations make your practice more engaging and rewarding.

PRACTICAL STEPS FOR ENGAGING WITH A CHAIR YOGA COMMUNITY

- **Join a Class:** Start with local or online classes to gain experience and meet others.
- **Participate in Online Groups:** Engage with social media communities, forums, and wellness apps for ideas and support.
- **Attend Workshops:** Explore local or virtual events to expand your practice.
- **Host Your Own Group:** Organize sessions with friends or neighbors, either in person or online.
- **Stay Connected:** Share your progress, celebrate milestones, and encourage others on their journey.

Final Thoughts

A supportive community transforms chair yoga from a solitary practice into a shared experience. Whether you join a class, engage online, or create your own group, these connections will enrich your journey and strengthen your commitment to health and wellness.

13

KEEP MOVING FORWARD

"Success is not final, failure is not fatal: It is the courage to continue that counts."

— WINSTON CHURCHILL

E very journey comes with challenges, and chair yoga is no exception. Some days, motivation will be high, and on other days, life will get in the way. But remember—**progress is built on consistency, not perfection**.

OVERCOMING OBSTACLES & STAYING MOTIVATED

It's easy to let stiffness, fatigue, or a busy schedule put exercising on the back burner. But the key to success is **adapting, not stopping**. Whether your challenge is mobility, self-doubt, or fear of injury, the solution is to start **small, stay consistent, and celebrate progress.**

- **Make it a habit:** Treat your chair yoga time like an important appointment—just 10 minutes a day can make a difference.
- **Track your progress:** Write down small victories, whether less stiffness, more flexibility, or improved confidence in daily movements.
- **Celebrate small wins:** Progress isn't just mastering a pose—it's feeling better, moving easier, and showing up for yourself.

BUILDING CONFIDENCE

Doubt is normal, but **your body is capable of growth and adaptation at any age**. Visualizing success, setting realistic goals, and connecting with a supportive community can help you stay committed. Remember:

- **You don't have to be perfect to make progress.**

- **You are stronger than you think.**
- **Every movement counts toward a healthier, more independent life.**

A REAL-LIFE REMINDER: YOU CAN DO THIS

I've seen firsthand how starting small—just **10 minutes of gentle movement each day**—can extend both the **quality and quantity** of life. My grandma remained active and joyful for many years because of her commitment to daily movement. Clients and patients well into their **late 90s**, who also made it a habit to do simple daily exercises, continued enjoying more quality time with their loved ones, hobbies, and recreational activities.

Their journeys—like yours—weren't about pushing through pain or expecting instant results. **They were about consistency, patience, and trusting the process.**

YOUR NEXT STEPS

Your chair yoga journey doesn't end here—it evolves. As you continue, remember:

- **Listen to your body:** Modify poses when needed, but don't be afraid to challenge yourself gradually.
- **Stay safe:** Use a stable chair, clear your space, and avoid overextending.

- **Keep going:** Each session is an investment in your health, mobility, and independence.

FINAL WORDS

Chair yoga isn't just about movement—it's about **building resilience, confidence, and a better quality of life**. Keep showing up, keep moving, and keep believing in yourself. You've got this!

CONCLUSION

"Movement is life. With every stretch and every step, we unlock the power to heal, to grow stronger, and to thrive—at any age."

— DR. YVETTE F

As we conclude this journey, it's time to reflect on the purpose that has guided us through each chapter: to help you cultivate strength, flexibility, and balance to enhance your quality of life. Chair yoga is more than a set of exercises—it's a powerful tool to maintain mobility, foster mindfulness, and empower yourself to live actively and independently.

By mastering foundational routines, connecting with supportive communities, and overcoming challenges, you've established a practice tailored to your needs. Each step—whether mastering a pose, integrating yoga into your daily routine, or celebrating milestones—demonstrates your resilience and commitment to self-care.

The greatest strength of chair yoga lies in its adaptability. Whether you practice the same 10-minute routine for a week or create your own routine with poses from two levels, every moment invested in your well-being matters. Your practice doesn't need to be perfect to be effective. The mindful movements, breaths, and moments of stillness you cultivate daily are cumulative steps toward better health and happiness.

As your abilities evolve, so can your practice. Revisit the routines and concepts in this book, adjusting them to your changing goals and challenges. Let your practice grow with you, supporting your physical and mental well-being throughout life.

CELEBRATE THE PROGRESS

Acknowledge how far you've come. Progress isn't always measured by dramatic leaps but by subtle improvements—feeling stronger, more balanced, or more at ease. Each time you show up for yourself, you affirm your dedication to living with vitality and grace. Celebrate these moments and let them fuel your continued growth.

SHARING THE JOY OF CHAIR YOGA

Your journey doesn't have to remain personal. Share the joy and benefits of chair yoga with friends, family, or your community. By introducing others to the practice or joining a group class, you can inspire those around you to prioritize their health and wellness.

Your story and experiences can motivate others to take their first steps toward better mobility, confidence, and well-being. Together, you can create a ripple effect of improved health and happiness.

LOOKING AHEAD

The end of this book is just the beginning of your chair yoga journey. With every breath, every pose, and every session, you are building a foundation for a healthier, more fulfilling life. Let this practice remind you of your ability to create positive change for yourself, one movement at a time.

Thank you for allowing me to be a part of your journey. Your dedication, curiosity, and openness are truly inspiring. As you move forward, embrace each session as an opportunity to nurture your body, mind, and spirit.

Here's to your continued strength, joy, and resilience. May chair yoga remain a source of empowerment and peace, for years to come.

BONUS 2: FREQUENTLY ASKED QUESTIONS & ANSWERS BY A PHYSICAL THERAPY DOCTOR

1. **Can these routines help me with urinary incontinence?** Yes! These routines were designed to strengthen from the center out. Just doing the core routines alone can and will strengthen all muscles responsible for bladder control. With regular practice engaging the pelvic floor muscles first, followed by the core muscles while performing knee extensions and alternating knee raises, you can improve urinary control. If you have concerns, consult with your healthcare provider for personalized guidance.

2. **How can I do these routines without aggravating my arthritic shoulder?** If you have arthritis in your shoulder, it's important to modify movements to avoid pain. The poses to be aware of are the reaching

ones. Choose gentle, pain-free ranges of motion when attempting these. Avoid forcing movements that cause discomfort, and use slow, controlled motions.

3. **I had a total hip replacement. Can chair yoga help?** Absolutely! Chair yoga can be a safe and effective way to regain flexibility, strength, and mobility after a hip replacement. Seated movements reduce stress on your hip joint while allowing you to work on posture, core stability, and lower body strength. Gentle exercises such as seated marching and controlled leg extensions can help maintain hip function without overloading the joint. Be sure to follow your surgeon's or physical therapist's guidelines for safe movement post-surgery.

4. **I am 90 years old. How can chair yoga improve my strength and flexibility?** Muscle can gain strength and flexibility at any age. These routines are designed to improve age-related muscle weakness and stiffness by engaging core, arm, and leg muscles through various adaptable poses. Through repetition, muscle strength and flexibility will improve, and you will know this when certain movements begin to feel easier and require less effort.

5. **I am afraid of falling but need to start exercising again. How do these routines improve my balance?** Fear of falling is common, but avoiding movement

can lead to further weakness and instability. These routines provide a secure way to rebuild strength and confidence in your balance. The routines focus on core engagement, postural awareness, and lower-body stability—key factors in fall prevention. Exercises such as seated marching and knee extensions train your body to respond better to balance challenges, reducing the risk of falls over time. As you progress through the three balance routines, you will begin to experience better body awareness and body control in all positions.

6. **Can chair yoga help with back pain?** Yes! Unless you have severe spinal conditions, chair yoga can help alleviate back pain by improving posture, strengthening core muscles, and increasing spine flexibility. A combination of progressed core stabilization and hip and spine flexibility poses found in these routines is instrumental in reducing and managing back pain.

7. **Will chair yoga help with circulation issues in my legs?** Definitely. Chair yoga encourages gentle movement, which can help stimulate circulation and reduce swelling in the legs. Exercises that involve seated leg lifts, knee extensions, and gentle stretching can improve blood flow and prevent stiffness. Consistent practice may also support vascular health and reduce discomfort related to poor circulation.

8. **What if I have limited mobility or use a wheelchair?** Chair yoga can be adapted for various mobility levels, including those who use wheelchairs. You can complete the routines sitting in your wheelchair. Many poses can be modified so you can participate comfortably and safely. The focus remains on improving posture, breathing, and gentle movement to promote flexibility, strength, and relaxation without needing to stand.

9. **How can I tell if the discomfort I feel when doing chair yoga poses is good or bad?** Discomfort is a common part of any new exercise program, especially when stretching muscles that have become tight or engaging muscles that haven't been used in a while. However, it's important to distinguish between productive discomfort and pain to avoid injury.

Mild Discomfort (Good Discomfort)—When holding a pose, you may feel a gentle stretch or muscle fatigue. This should ease up once you release the position or take a break. This type of discomfort is normal and often a sign that your muscles are adapting and getting stronger or more flexible.

Pain (Bad Discomfort) – If discomfort turns into sharp, stabbing, burning, or shooting pain—especially if it radiates down your arm or leg—this could indicate a nerve, joint, or muscle issue. If modifying your positioning does not relieve it, stop that pose immediately and avoid it until you determine the cause.

Overstretching and Muscle Fatigue—A stretch should feel gentle and relieving, not painful. If you push too far, the discomfort can quickly become pain, signaling that you're overstretching. Similarly, holding a pose too long may cause excessive muscle fatigue, leading to pain or cramping. Always stop before discomfort turns into pain.

If pain persists after your session or worsens over time, it's a sign that you may need to modify your routine further or consult a healthcare professional. Listen to your body, and remember—yoga should feel good, not painful.

10. Are there any risks associated with chair yoga? Chair yoga is generally very safe, but like any form of exercise, there are risks if movements are done incorrectly. To minimize risks:

- Use a stable chair
- Move slowly and mindfully
- Avoid overstretching or forcing movements
- Keep feet flat on the floor for balance

PLEASE LEAVE YOUR AMAZON REVIEW!

I am deeply honored to have been your guide on this journey toward progressive **strength, stability, and movement**. I may never know how many lives this book will impact, but my hope and prayer is that it reaches as many people as possible.

Your Review Matters!

By leaving a review, you help **others discover this resource** and make it more accessible to those who need it most. If you haven't already, please take a moment to support this mission by leaving a review on Amazon now.

Go to this link:
https://a.co/d/ggZBQ6S
Or scan this QR code with your phone camera:

1. Click on the **review ratings** and select the "**Write a Review**" button.
2. Share a few sentences about the part of the book you liked the most.
3. Take a picture of your favorite page, quote, or book cover, and upload it to your review.
4. Title your review.
5. Press the yellow "**Submit**" button.

With gratitude,
Movement Freedom Publications

REFERENCES

Effect of chair yoga therapy on functional fitness and health. *National Center for Biotechnology Information.* Retrieved from https://www.ncbi.nlm.nih.gov/pmc/articles/PMC10094373/

3 misconceptions and 3 fun facts about chair yoga. *Rise and Vibe Yoga.* Retrieved from https://www.riseandvibeyoga.com/blog/chair-yoga

What chair is good for chair yoga? *Flow With Me.* Retrieved from https://www.flowithme.com/post/what-chair-is-good-for-chair-yoga

Yoga props, clothing, and accessories. *AARP.* Retrieved from https://www.aarp.org/health/healthy-living/info-2017/yoga-clothes-props-photo.html

How to create a senior-friendly exercise space at home. *Senior Helpers.* Retrieved from https://www.seniorhelpers.com/or/corvallis/resources/blogs/2023-07-17/

The best free online yoga classes for older adults. *Nice News.* Retrieved from https://nicenews.com/health-and-wellness/best-free-yoga-classes-for-seniors/

Chair yoga for seniors: Benefits and poses for beginners. *Medical News Today.* Retrieved from https://www.medicalnewstoday.com/articles/chair-yoga-for-seniors

Chair yoga for seniors with limited mobility. *Banner Health.* Retrieved from https://www.bannerhealth.com/healthcareblog/teach-me/chair-yoga-gentle-exercises-for-seniors-with-limited-mobility

Why proper posture is imperative for seniors. *ASC Care.* Retrieved from https://www.asccare.com/why-proper-posture-is-imperative-for-seniors/

Finding balance: How yoga supports healthy aging. *MBK Senior Living.* Retrieved from https://www.mbkseniorliving.com/senior-living/wa/bellevue/the-bellettini/mbk-blog?article=finding-balance-how-yoga-supports-healthy-aging-for-seniors

Arthritis-friendly yoga poses. *Arthritis Foundation.* Retrieved from https://www.arthritis.org/health-wellness/healthy-living/physical-activity/yoga/arthritis-friendly-yoga

6 best balance exercises for seniors to improve stability. *Silver Sneakers.* Retrieved from https://www.silversneakers.com/blog/balance-exercises-seniors/

Yoga after hip replacement. *Joint Replacement Hawaii.* Retrieved from https://www.jointreplacementhawaii.com/yoga-after-hip-replacement/

LeBlanc, A. D., & Evans, H. J. (1990). Muscle atrophy and muscle fiber loss: The first week of bed rest. *Journal of Applied Physiology.* Retrieved from https://pubmed.ncbi.nlm.nih.gov/2197699/

15 tips for creating an amazing home yoga studio. *Yoga Basics.* Retrieved from https://www.yogabasics.com/connect/yoga-blog/home-yoga-studio/

Exercise and physical activity worksheets. *National Institute on Aging.* Retrieved from https://www.nia.nih.gov/health/exercise-and-physical-activity/exercise-and-physical-activity-worksheets

Try yoga at work with these 7 chair yoga poses. *YouAligned.* Retrieved from https://youaligned.com/yoga-at-work-chair-yoga-poses/

Mindfulness-based interventions for older adults. *National Center for Biotechnology Information.* Retrieved from https://www.ncbi.nlm.nih.gov/pmc/articles/PMC4868399/

Chair yoga for stress relief: Techniques to calm your mind. *Amanda Stivers.* Retrieved from https://www.amandastivers.com/blog/chair-yoga-for-stress-relief

Yoga impacts cognitive health. *National Center for Biotechnology Information.* Retrieved from https://www.ncbi.nlm.nih.gov/pmc/articles/PMC10033324/

How yoga can ease pain and improve mobility. *Brain & Life.* Retrieved from https://www.brainandlife.org/articles/experts-say-yoga-can-ease-pain-and-improve-mobility-for

Confidence and positive attitude help older adults stick with exercise. *Human Kinetics.* Retrieved from https://us.humankinetics.com/blogs/excerpt/confidence-and-positive-attitude-help-older-adults-stick-with-exercise

Yoga as a fall prevention strategy. *Stoughton Health.* Retrieved from https://stoughtonhealth.com/yoga-as-a-fall-prevention-strategy/

Adaptive yoga: Making yoga accessible for every body. *Healthline.* Retrieved from https://www.healthline.com/health/fitness/adaptive-yoga

Discover 29 chair yoga innovations for 2024. *Place Ideal.* Retrieved from https://placeideal.com/discover-29-chair-yoga-innovations-for-2024-accessible-modern-practices/

How technology supports seniors' fitness programs. *Seaton Senior Living.* Retrieved from https://www.seatonseniorliving.com/senior-living-blog/how-technology-supports-seniors-fitness-programs/

Office yoga poses: Examples and benefits. *EAP Employee Wellness.* Retrieved from https://eapemployeewellness.com/corporate-yoga/office-yoga-poses/

Feuerstein, G. (2001). The yoga tradition: Its history, literature, philosophy and practice. Prescott, AZ: Hohm Press. Retrieved from https://www.hohmpress.com/products/the-yoga-tradition-paperback

Saraswati, S. S. (2008). *Asana Pranayama Mudra Bandha* (4th ed.). Bihar, India: Yoga Publications Trust. Retrieved fromMy Book

Movement Freedom Publications. (2024). *Top Ten Benefits of Orthopedic Physical Therapy for Seniors.* Published by Movement Freedom Publications. Retrieved fromMy Book

Made in the USA
Coppell, TX
03 July 2025

51409318R10095